NEUROSCIENCE RESEARCH PROGRESS

ADVANCES IN NEUROIMAGING RESEARCH

NEUROSCIENCE RESEARCH PROGRESS

Additional books in this series can be found on Nova's website
under the Series tab.

Additional e-books in this series can be found on Nova's website
under the e-book tab.

NEUROSCIENCE RESEARCH PROGRESS

ADVANCES IN NEUROIMAGING RESEARCH

VICTORIA ASHER-HANSLEY
EDITOR

New York

Library of Congress Cataloging-in-Publication Data

ISBN: 978-1-63321-307-4

Library of Congress Control Number: 2014942200

Published by Nova Science Publishers, Inc. † New York

Contents

Preface

This book discusses neural correlation between reading deficits in individuals with developmental dyslexia. It also includes topics on electrical imaging in neuropsychiatry; prenatal magnetic resonance imaging of the brain and spine; and normal pressure hydrocephalus.

Chapter I – Neuroimaging has had an enormous impact on the way human cognition is studied *in vivo*. With the advent of fMRI, scientists have been able to ask questions regarding individual differences which could not have been addressed with PET. These, are particularly important for studying developmental disorders, such as dyslexia because research suggests that participants with dyslexia (DPs) form a heterogeneous population. There are three main theories of dyslexia: the phonological (PDT), visual magnocellular (MDT) and cerebellar (CDT). The majority of neuroimaging studies, motivated by these theories, have shortcomings. First, they have relied on group comparisons which can obscure the less frequent differences between DPs and controls (CPs). Second, they mostly tested one underlying cause, postulated by one theory. Third, the majority of them focused on detecting a deficit without empirically demonstrating its relationship with reading deficit which defines this disorder. The goal of this research is to shed more light on the neural correlates of reading deficit in dyslexia and address these criticisms First, by using a multiple case study to investigate individual differences among DPs. Such comparisons would not have been possible with PET. Second, by contrasting the predictions, of each of the main theories, on the neural correlates of the reading impairment in one sample of DPs. The behavioural studies suggest that there are subtypes of dyslexia, however, they cannot be tested by focusing on one theory. Third, by using a reading task and fMRI - which provides an opportunity for directly testing the relationship between the predictions of a given theory and the neural correlates of reading impairment. Eighteen individual DPs and 16 CPs were tested in a multiple case study. Participants were right-handed, with native English, normal vision and hearing and without clinical ADHD and DCD. To ensure that no confounds were present due to differences between a DP and CPs in IQ, handedness and age, these were entered into the analysis as covariates. The neuroimaging task involved silent reading of individual words and fixating on a cross (baseline) in an event-related design. Four findings were revealed. First, the neural correlates of reading deficit in dyslexia in all cases, except one, are consistent with the predictions of the PDT and CDT, in one case with the visual MDT and in ten cases with a hypothetical visual (not magnocellular) deficit theory; most cases are consistent with more than one theory. Second, there are considerable individual differences in the neural correlates of reading deficit. Even where they are consistent with the same theory in two DPs, the areas can differ. Third, the results reveal that the lack of deficit on a behavioural test does not mean that the neural correlates of reading are intact. Fourth, a large number of DPs who have a similar profile on the behavioural measures exhibited dissimilar profiles on the neural level. These findings suggest that endophenotypes uncovered by neuroimaging will enable researchers to find important links between the behavioural and genetic characteristics of DPs. Multidisciplinary research on individual differences, including neuroimaging, behavioural and genetic measures within a multiple-deficit model holds significant promise.

Chapter II – Quantitative Electroencephalography (QEEG) combined with Low Resolution Electro-magnetic Tomography Analysis (QEEG/LORETA) is a relatively new form of functional imaging which is able to indicate which region of the brain is malfunctioning and contributing to a patient's symptoms. In contrast to functional MRI, PET and SPECT imaging, which measure secondary metabolic processes, QEEG/LORETA records direct neuronal activity through the surface of the head. Introduction of QEEG/LORETA brain imaging has improved our diagnostic ability in neuropsychiatric practice by identifying dysregulated cortical areas implicated in patient's symptoms. Additional use of LORETA Z-score neurofeedback (NFB) enables us to directly target these areas of dysregulation in order to improve associated symptoms. Based on approximately 250 patients treated in our clinic with Z-score LORETA NFB, a detailed analysis of selected cases is presented. Cases include depression/anxiety, chronic pain, epilepsy, ADHD and cognitive dysfunction. Specific areas of dysregulation attributed to particular conditions identified by LORETA are presented: Anterior Cingulate and Insular cortex in pain syndromes; as well as specific Brodmann's Areas in other cases. Follow up findings of QEEG/LORETA electrical imaging after NFB and computerized cognitive testing are discussed. In addition, cases of Z-score LORETA NFB mediated cognitive enhancement are shown. This chapter encompasses examples of the application of functional neurology in neuropsychiatry.

Chapter III – Fetal magnetic resonance (MR) imaging is an increasingly available technique used to evaluate the fetal brain and spine. This has become possible due to recent advances in technology and advances in coil design, making this diagnostic tool applicable in pregnant women with low risks to the mother and fetus. This provides a unique opportunity to evaluate processes that cannot be approached by any other current imaging technique and affords a unique opportunity for studying in vivo brain development and early diagnosis of congenital abnormalities inadequately visualized or undetectable by prenatal sonography. The authors discuss briefly about technical features like utility, application and safety and focus mainly on normal fetal brain development, role of fetal MR imaging in the evaluation of fetal ventriculomegaly, brain abnormalities such as of the corpus callosum, malformations of cortical development and spine abnormalities, such as spinal dysraphism. They present the medical and economical impact of such diagnostic modality and also discuss some challenges and advances towards future outcomes.

Chapter IV – Normal pressure hydrocephalus (NPH) is a condition characterized by gait disturbance, dementia and/or urinary incontinence without causative disorders, as well as dilation of ventricular system due to disturbance of cerebrospinal fluid (CSF) circulation with normal CSF pressure and no secondary cause˙ It is a differential diagnosis for most of the dementia syndromes and occurs mainly in elderly populations. Neuroimaging is fundamental not only in affirming diagnosis with anatomical patterns, but also increasing evidence points to qualitative and quantitative measures which are important to perform differential diagnosis with simultaneous diseases like Alzheimer disease and vascular dementia. Magnetic resonance imaging (MRI) and functional neuroimaging techniques like Positron Emission Tomography (PET) and Single Photon Emission Tomography (SPECT) are being employed to evaluate cerebrospinal fluid biomarkers and periventricular hemodynamic parameters in order to better classify those patients and predict their response to provocative tests and to shunt procedures. The authors discuss the main current aspects and new protocols towards management of NPH.

In: Advances in Neuroimaging Research
Editor: Victoria Asher-Hansley

ISBN: 978-1-63321-307-4

Chapter I

An fMRI Multiple Case Study of the Neural Correlates of Reading Deficit in Individuals with Developmental Dyslexia: Theoretical Implications

*Agnieszka Anna Reid**
School of Life and Health Sciences,
Aston University, Birmingham, UK

Abstract

Neuroimaging has had an enormous impact on the way human cognition is studied *in vivo*. With the advent of fMRI, scientists have been able to ask questions regarding individual differences which could not have been addressed with PET. These, are particularly important for studying developmental disorders, such as dyslexia because research suggests that participants with dyslexia (DPs) form a heterogeneous population. There are three main theories of dyslexia: the phonological (PDT), visual magnocellular (MDT) and cerebellar (CDT). The majority of neuroimaging studies, motivated by these theories, have shortcomings. First, they have relied on group comparisons which can obscure the less frequent differences between DPs and controls (CPs). Second, they mostly tested one underlying cause, postulated by one theory. Third, the majority of them focused on detecting a deficit without empirically demonstrating its relationship with reading deficit which defines this disorder. The goal of this research is to shed more light on the neural correlates of reading deficit in dyslexia and address these criticisms First, by using a multiple case study to investigate individual differences among DPs. Such comparisons would not have been possible with PET. Second, by contrasting the predictions, of each of the main theories, on the neural correlates of the reading impairment in one sample of DPs. The behavioural studies suggest that there are subtypes

* Corresponding author: Dr. Agnieszka A. Reid. 41 Corrie Road, Cambridge, CB1-3QP, UK. E-mail: agnieszka.reid @virginmedia.com.

of dyslexia, however, they cannot be tested by focusing on one theory. Third, by using a reading task and fMRI - which provides an opportunity for directly testing the relationship between the predictions of a given theory and the neural correlates of reading impairment. Eighteen individual DPs and 16 CPs were tested in a multiple case study. Participants were right-handed, with native English, normal vision and hearing and without clinical ADHD and DCD. To ensure that no confounds were present due to differences between a DP and CPs in IQ, handedness and age, these were entered into the analysis as covariates. The neuroimaging task involved silent reading of individual words and fixating on a cross (baseline) in an event-related design. Four findings were revealed. First, the neural correlates of reading deficit in dyslexia in all cases, except one, are consistent with the predictions of the PDT and CDT, in one case with the visual MDT and in ten cases with a hypothetical visual (not magnocellular) deficit theory; most cases are consistent with more than one theory. Second, there are considerable individual differences in the neural correlates of reading deficit. Even where they are consistent with the same theory in two DPs, the areas can differ. Third, the results reveal that the lack of deficit on a behavioural test does not mean that the neural correlates of reading are intact. Fourth, a large number of DPs who have a similar profile on the behavioural measures exhibited dissimilar profiles on the neural level. These findings suggest that endophenotypes uncovered by neuroimaging will enable researchers to find important links between the behavioural and genetic characteristics of DPs. Multidisciplinary research on individual differences, including neuroimaging, behavioural and genetic measures within a multiple-deficit model holds significant promise.

Keywords: Dyslexia, fMRI, multiple-case study, reading, comorbidity

Introduction

Neuroimaging methods have had an enormous impact on the way human cognition is studied *in vivo* in health and disease. With the advent of fMRI, scientists have been able to ask questions which could not have been addressed with PET, such as questions to do with individual differences. These, are particularly important for studying developmental disorders, such as developmental dyslexia (henceforth dyslexia) because recent behavioural research (Heim et al., 2008; Menghini et al., 2010; Ramus et al., 2003; Reid, Szczerbinski, Iskierka-Kasperek, and Hansen, 2007; Snowling, 2008) suggests that participants with dyslexia (DPs) form a heterogeneous population.

Dyslexia is a prevalent, specific, childhood disorder the symptoms of which persist throughout the entire life-span of an individual. According to the definition approved by the British Dyslexia Association in October 2007, "dyslexia is a specific learning difficulty that mainly affects the development of literacy and language related skills. It is likely to be present at birth and to be life-long in its effects. It is characterised by difficulties with phonological processing, rapid naming, working memory, processing speed and the automatic development of skills that may not be consistent with an individual's other cognitive abilities. It tends to be resistant to conventional teaching methods, but its effect can be mitigated by appropriate, specific intervention, including the application of information technology and supportive counselling" (British Dyslexia Association, 2007).

The prevalence rates for dyslexia range from 5 to 17.5% (Shaywitz, 1998). Some researchers have indicated that dyslexia occurs more often in males than in females.

Nevertheless, such an outcome could also result from referral bias (Habib, 2000; Shaywitz et al., 2003). A more recent publication (Rutter et al., 2004), however, demonstrated that in four independent epidemiological studies the rates of reading disability were significantly higher in boys than in girls.

1.1. Dyslexia As a Broader Phenotype

The difficulties experienced by participants with dyslexia (DPs) are not usually limited to difficulties in the development of literacy and language related skills and the aforementioned cognitive abilities. Difficulties with distinguishing between right and left (Miles, 1993), temporal sequencing (learning to tell the time, remembering days of the week, months, etc.) (Miles, 1993), planning and organization (Brunswick, 2011) and poor spatial sequencing (Stein and Walsh, 1997), may also occur, to mention just a few. The key issue here is the extent to which non-literacy deficits found in dyslexia are part of the broader dyslexia syndrome and to what extent they are related to the other developmental disorders which co-occur with dyslexia.

1.2. Findings from Behavioural and Molecular Genetics

Dyslexia is characterised by a strong heritable component (Poelmans, Buitelaar, Pauls, and Franke, 2011). The findings from behavioural and molecular genetics are important because they shape the understanding of this disorder (and its co-occurrence with other developmental disorders). Hallgren (1950) and Thomas (1905) noted that dyslexia runs in families, implicating a genetic basis, however, this is not sufficient, because co-occurrence of literacy problems can result from a shared environment.

Hence, scientists started to study MZ (Monozygotic) twins, who have almost identical genetic material, and DZ (Dizygotic) twins who share approximately half their genes. Both types of twins are assumed to share the same environment (there is also non-shared environment within and outside a family, which refers to the variance not accounted for by shared environment or by heredity, it also includes error measurement (Plomin, DeFries, McClearn, and McGuffin, 2008)). If MZ twins' reading ability (on the populational level) is more similar than DZ twins' reading ability (on the populational level), it suggests that genetic factors play a role in reading ability. Such a pattern of results was found in a study carried out in the Colorado Learning Disabilities Research Centre. A concordance rate (identity of traits within twins) for dyslexia of 38% in DZ twins, as compared to 68% in MZ twins was reported (DeFries, Fulker, and LaBuda, 1987), which suggests that genetic influence is of moderate importance (DeFries and Alarcon, 1996).

One problem with a method which relies on concordance rates is that it is best for studying traits which are categorical. Because DPs are characterised by reading problems which vary in degree, DeFries and Fulker (1985) developed a method which deals with continuous traits in twins. Using this method with DPs, the authors reported an estimated group heritability of approximately 50%; this means that 50% of the difference in reading scores between the general population and the probands can be accounted for by genetic differences. However, heritability seems to be higher in children with higher IQs (Olson,

Datta, and DeFries, 1999) and in children who have more serious reading problems (Bishop, 2001). These findings, therefore suggest that genetic influence may be stronger in some subgroups of DPs than in other subgroups.

Relatively recently, molecular genetics started a new chapter on the identification of genes implicated in dyslexia and so far fifteen such genes have been suggested by cytogenetic findings, linkage and association studies. These include: *DYX1C1* on the longer arm of chromosome 15 (15q21) (Taipale et al., 2003); *KIAA0319* (Cope et al., 2005; Francks et al., 2004), *DCDC2* (Meng et al., 2005), *THEM2* (Deffenbacher et al., 2004), *TTRAP* (Deffenbacher et al., 2004; Francks et al., 2004; Meng et al., 2005) and *VMP* (Londin, Meng, and Gruen, 2003) on the shorter arm of chromosome 6 (6p22); *ROBO1* on the shorter arm of chromosome 3 (3p12) (Hannula-Jouppi et al., 2005); *C2ORF3* and *MROL19* on the shorter arm of chromosome 2 (2p12-p16) (Anthoni et al., 2007); *KIAA0319L* on the short arm of chromosome 1 (1p35) (Couto et al., 2008); *S100B* and *DIP2A,* on the longer arm of chromosome 21 (21q22.3) (Poelmans et al., 2009); *FMR1* on the longer arm of chromosome X (Xq27) (de Kovel et al., 2004) and on the longer arm of chromosome 7 - *GTF2I* (7q11.23) (Antonell et al., 2010; Meyer-Lindenberg, Mervis, and Berman, 2006) and *DOCK4* (7q31.1) (Pagnamenta et al., 2010).

More recently, three novel dyslexia candidate genes (from known linkage regions) were proposed (Poelmans et al., 2011). These included: *SLIT2* on the shorter arm of chromosome 4 (4p15.32) (Bates et al., 2007); *HMGB1* on the longer arm of chromosome 13 (13q12.3) (Igo et al., 2006) and *VAPA* on the shorter arm of chromosome 18 (18p11.2) (Bates et al., 2007; Fisher, Francks, Marlow et al., 2002). Four other genes, associated with dyslexia and reading deficit, have also been reported. These include *ATP2C2* and *CMIP* on chromosome 16 and *FOXP2* and *CNTNAP2* on chromosome 7 (Kaminen et al., 2003; MacDermot et al., 2005; Peter et al., 2011; Scerri et al., 2011; Wilcke et al., 2012). *DCDC2*, *KIAA0319*, *DYX1C1*, *FOXP2* and *CNTNAP2* are the most studied genes.

Interestingly, molecular genetic findings point to abnormal connectivity in dyslexia. The roles of genes implicated in dyslexia were investigated, among others, in RAN interference (RANi) studies with animals. For instance, the results revealed that *DYX1C1* (Rosen et al., 2007; Wang et al., 2006), *KIAA0319* (Paracchini et al., 2006) and *DCDC2* (Burbridge et al., 2008; Meng et al., 2005) are involved in neuronal migration. *ROBO1* has been implicated in axon growth (Zhu, Li, Zhou, Wu, and Rao, 1999). More recently, six new genes (*KIAA0319L*, *S100B*, *DOCK4*, *FMR1*, *DIP2A* and *GTF2I*), implicated in dyslexia, have been reported to be involved in neuronal migration and neurite outgrowth.

A theory where neural migration deficit is the underlying cause of dyslexia has been proposed (Galaburda, 2005; Galaburda, LoTurco, Ramus, Fitch, and Rosen, 2006). According to this theory, impaired neuronal migration causes ectopias and microgyri which tend to agglomerate most densely within the L perisylvian cortex and this in turn causes dyslexia. However, as the authors have pointed out, the genes implicated so far in dyslexia appear to have a general function in neuronal migration and guidance, so are unlikely to restrict migration to these specific areas. Some additional mechanisms may be involved to restrict neuronal migration to certain brain areas, or the migration deficit may be more general in nature affecting many more areas throughout the brain, including for instance the V5/MT and the cerebellum.

Linkage studies suggest that more 'dyslexia genes' will be identified. There are at least two reasons for this. First, although, a single gene mutation may be associated with dyslexia, as with *ROBO1*, such cases should be rare because it is a heterogeneous disorder and therefore it is likely that most cases will be associated with several susceptibility alleles, each contributing a portion to an individual's risk of developing this disorder (Fisher, 2006). It is possible that there are a large number of such genes and their dyslexia susceptibility may be frequent in the general population and there may be large numbers of possible combinations of alleles conferring a high susceptibility to dyslexia. Second, behavioural findings point to the fact that dyslexia is a heterogeneous developmental disorder and even within a given cognitive subtype of dyslexia, several genotypes may be compatible with it. For instance, many genes are involved in neural migration, and therefore neuronal migration can be potentially affected in a similar way by many different genes.

1.3. Dyslexia and Comorbidity with Other Developmental Disorders

There is now considerable evidence that dyslexia co-occurs more frequently than would be expected by chance with other developmental disorders such as ADHD (Attention Deficit Hyperactivity Disorder) and Developmental Coordination Disorder (DCD). Heritability estimates for ADHD range from 60-80% (Smalley, 1997). Approximately 25-40% of children with ADHD or dyslexia also have another developmental disorder (August and GarWnkel, 1990; Carroll, Maughan, Goodman, and Meltzer, 2005; Dykman and Ackerman, 1991; Semrud-Clikeman et al., 1992; Willcutt and Pennington, 2000). Kaplan, Wilson, Dewey and Crawford (1998) revealed that 42% of their reading disabled children also met the criteria for ADHD.

The finding that dyslexia co-occurs more frequently than would be expected by chance with ADHD (Pennington, 2006) and with other developmental disorders, such as DCD, implies that dyslexia and ADHD are not completely independent disorders. Results from cognitive, behavioural and molecular genetic studies lend some support for this view. Evidence was found for speed of processing being a cognitive risk factor which is shared by both ADHD and dyslexia (Shanahan et al., 2006). Behavioural genetic studies (Light, Pennington, Gilger, and DeFries, 1995; Stevenson, Pennington, Gilger, DeFries, and Gillis, 2006; Willcutt, Pennington, and DeFries, 2000) have reported bivariate heritability for reading disorder and ADHD. However, results from molecular genetic studies are less straightforward. For instance, a pioneering study on ADHD and reading comorbidity found that the dyslexia risk locus on chromosome 6p22 is also implicated in ADHD (Willcutt et al., 2002). Although, a more recent study (Couto et al., 2009) revealed a strong association for both inattention, as well as hyperactivity and impulsivity subtypes of ADHD for the markers in the 6p22 region, it found no overlap for ADHD and reading skills markers. This may be because only 31 individuals with ADHD, out of 264 probands and 55 siblings were diagnosed with reading disability. Loo et al. (2004) reported common loci on chromosome 16p, 17q and possibly on 10p contributing to both reading measures and ADHD. The findings for 16p and 17q replicated earlier findings for the same data set (Fisher, Francks, McCracken et al., 2002; Ogdie et al., 2003; Smalley et al., 2002). Finally, Doyle et al. (2008) reported a region on chromosome 3 (3q13) which exhibited a suggestive linkage with the inattention subtype of ADHD and a range of neurocognitive traits. Interestingly, 3q13 overlaps with the region which contains the *ROBO1* gene associated with dyslexia (Nopola-Hemmi et al., 2001).

DCD (also known as dyspraxia) is a marked impairment in the development of motor coordination. It has been estimated that approximately 6% of 5-11 year old children have this disorder (American Psychiatric Association, 1994). There is growing evidence that some reading impaired individuals exhibit motor difficulties (Denckla, 1985; Fawcett and Nicholson, 1995; Haslum, 1989; Iversen, Berg, Ellertsen, and Tonnessen, 2005; McPhillips and Sheehy, 2004; Miles, 1993; Wolff, Cohen, and Drake, 1984). The prevalence of dyslexia and DCD comorbidity was assessed to be 63% in Kaplan et al.'s (1998) sample. However, comorbidity depends on the characteristics of the reference sample. DCD in dyslexia is not the same as dyslexia in DCD. To date no genetic overlap has been reported for dyslexia and DCD (Pennington and Bishop, 2009).

1.4. Current Main Theories of the Underlying Cause of Dyslexia

Although the current thinking about dyslexia is changing, especially in the light of the findings from behavioural and molecular genetics (Pennington, 2006; 2011), there have been and still currently are three main causal theories of dyslexia: the Phonological Deficit Theory (PDT) (Bradley and Bryant, 1983; Paulesu et al., 1996; Ramus et al., 2003; Shaywitz et al., 1998; Snowling, 2000; Vellutino, 1979), the visual Magnocellular Deficit Theory (MDT) (Hansen, Stein, Orde, Winter, and Talcott, 2001; Lovegrove et al., 1982; Stein, 2001; 2003; Stein and Talcott, 1999; Stein, Talcott, and Witton, 2001; Stein and Walsh, 1997) and the Cerebellar Deficit Theory (CDT) (Fawcett and Nicolson, 1999; Nicolson and Fawcett, 1990; Nicolson and Fawcett, 2008; Nicolson et al., 1999; Nicolson, Fawcett, and Dean, 2001). Each theory postulates a different underlying cause of literacy difficulties in dyslexia. Each theory also predicts a different set of associated difficulties; these difficulties may be linked to a reading deficit, but not necessarily (please see below).

Morton and Frith (1995) proposed that it is helpful to make a distinction between different levels of explanation within a given theory. The authors proposed: 1) the biological level and the environmental level (where search for causes and cures take place), 2) the behavioural level (where assessments and observations are recorded) and 3) the cognitive level (where a disorder is presented as a recognizable and distinct entity, in spite of variable symptoms).

1.4.1. The Phonological Deficit Theory

The PDT was formulated first on the cognitive level. According to the PDT (Frith, 1999; Lundberg and Hoien, 2001; Rack, Snowling, and Olson, 1992; Ramus et al., 2003; Snowling, 2000; Snowling and Caravolas, 2007; Vellutino, Fletcher, Snowling, and Scanlon, 2004) *phonological deficit* is the underlying cause of dyslexia on the cognitive level. This means that DPs have a specific impairment in the representation and processing of speech sounds (phonemes) (Snowling, 2000; Snowling and Caravolas, 2007). According to this theory, the phonological deficit leads to poor grapheme-phoneme conversion (defined as a process which is required when pseudowords are presented visually and have to be recognised in the auditory modality (Snowling, 1980)) and this in turn leads to poor reading (as measured by reading tests on the behavioural level).

It is claimed that the phonological deficit also manifests itself on the behavioural level by difficulties in: phonological awareness (Bradley and Bryant, 1983; Olson, Wise, Conners,

Rack, and Fulker, 1989; Ramus et al., 2003), phonological fluency (naming tasks) (Denckla and Rudel, 1976; Paulesu et al., 2001; Ramus et al., 2003; Reid et al., 2007) and verbal short-term memory (Brady, Shankweiler, and Mann, 1983; Paulesu et al., 2000; Ramus et al., 2003). According to Frith (1997) the underlying cause of dyslexia on the biological level is abnormality within the perisylvian brain region. This issue will be discussed in more detail in the section on neuroimaging studies presented below.

More recently the PDT has been updated (Hulme and Snowling, 2009), building on the older version of the PDT (Frith, 1997), with a few adjustments. First, a genetic level was added to the biological level. The authors focused on genes on chromosomes 6, 15 and 18, arguing that they affect the development of the L hemisphere brain networks and especially the development of the temporo-parietal cortex. Second, also on the biological level, the term 'perisylvian region' was replaced with 'L temporo-parietal' and 'L frontal' regions. Third, as in the older model (Frith, 1997) brain abnormalities were hypothesised to lead to a reading deficit through the phonological deficit; however in the updated model it is hypothesised that reading deficit could also be caused by "language delay" which leads to phonological deficit. According to the updated version of the PDT a more severe phonological deficit leads to more severe reading difficulties and feedback to reduce brain activity in areas subserving phonological processing and reading.

1.4.2. The Magnocellular Deficit Theory

The visual MDT (Hansen et al., 2001; Stein, 2003; Stein and Kapoula, 2012; Stein and Walsh, 1997) claims that the underlying cause of literacy problems in dyslexia is not language specific, but a more general impairment of the visual magnocellular system (which is specialised for processing fast temporal visual information) with spared parvocellular system. Magnocellular cells are characterised by thick myelination and rapidly conducting axons. They have greater dendritic area which allows them to get information from an area of the retina ten times larger than that for parvocells. They respond best to lower spatial frequencies but they have a contrast sensitivity, luminance and temporal sensitivity ten times higher than parvocells. The MDT was the first to propose a route from the biological level to the cognitive level.

Magnocellular neurons are defined at the level of the retinal ganglion cell (conveying the output from the retina), which have specific projections to LGN. Magnocellular cells have large receptive fields and respond relatively transiently to sustained illumination; they are able to follow rapid changes in stimulus. They are therefore concerned with the movement of a stimulus and its gross features (Tessier-Lavigne, 2000).

The magnocellular pathway is characterised by a hierarchical nature of anatomical connections (Albright, 1993). From the LGN, magnocellular neurons project to the primary visual (striate) cortex (V1) - first to layer 4Cα and then to layer 4B. Cells in layer 4B (which themselves are not magnocells) project directly to the V5/MT as well as to V2 (secondary – extrastriate visual cortex) from which cells also project to the V5/MT (Wurtz and Kandel, 2000). This is known as the magnocellular-dorsal pathway (Wurtz and Kandel, 2000). Motion sensitivity arises first in V1 and V2. However, in V1 and presumably in V2, only a small proportion of cells show motion sensitivity, and each cell is sensitive to motion in a small portion of the entire visual space (due to small receptive fields) (Wurtz and Kandel, 2000).

Motion detection across space relies on convergent output from V1 (and V2) to higher order regions, such as the V5/MT. V5/MT is hypothesised to be receiving the input predominantly from the magnocellular stream (Tootell and Taylor, 1995; Watson et al., 1993) and hence is usually the main target of investigations into the magnocellular system (e.g., Eden et al., 1996) (for more details please see the section 'Neuroimaging studies investigating visual magnocellular processing').

The results in support of the MDT include: unsteady binocular fixation (e.g., Stein, 2001), reduced contrast sensitivity (e.g., Lovegrove et al., 1982) and a significantly higher threshold for perception of coherent movement in random dot kinematograms in DPs than CPs (e.g., Hansen et al., 2001). For further details on the visual MDT please see the review by Stein and Walsh (1997) and for a critical review of the MDT see Skottun (2000).

From a developmental point of view, the MDT claims that the visual magnocellular system is impaired from birth and this impairment has a genetic origin. According to Stein (2001) the clearest genetic result is for linkage to the region on the short arm of chromosome 6 which helps to control the production of antibodies.

The magnocellular system is hypothesised to play an important role in reading and orthographic and phonological representations (Stein, 2001). First, it subserves the process of image stabilization and/or letter localization in words during reading (please see a study by Liederman et al. (2003) presented in the section 'Neuroimaging studies investigating visual magnocellular processing'); Second, visual magnocellular impairment affects orthographic knowledge, through reading skill. Third, the magnocellular system affects phonological representations through orthographic representations (Stein, 2001).

Because it is difficult to disentangle the orthographic from the phonological influences in reading, a number of experiments involving magnocellular function in reading and orthography have been performed on exception words (e.g., *pint* and *yacht*) and on Olson's pseudohomophone test (Olson et al., 1989). The processing of exception words, which cannot be read by assembling the constituent phonemes, biases towards orthographic processing. For instance, Talcott et al. (2000) reported that visual motion sensitivity explained independent variance in orthographic skill in unselected 10-year-old primary school children, after controlling for overall reading ability and IQ. Furthermore, in a study, which involved three hundred and fifty randomly selected primary school children (Talcott et al., 2002), visual motion sensitivity was a significant predictor of children's literacy skills and their orthographic and phonological skills.

1.4.3. The Cerebellar Deficit Theory

The CDT was originally formulated on the behavioural level as an automatization deficit theory (Nicolson and Fawcett, 1990). It is supported by the findings from a dual task paradigm, which involved balancing, defined as maintaining one's body in a state of equilibrium, while performing a secondary task. The results revealed that although under optimal conditions DPs could balance as well as CPs, in a dual task, DPs balanced significantly worse than the CPs (Nicolson and Fawcett, 1990). The authors suggested that one explanation of the results is that, unlike the CPs, DPs need to invest significant conscious effort for monitoring balance, and therefore their performance is significantly influenced by any secondary task which distracts attention from the primary task. This suggests that DPs' motor balance is poorly automatised. The authors concluded that it could be that DPs' reading problems are symptoms of the failure to fully automatize skills, which may be a more general learning deficit.

Subsequently, the automatization deficit theory was re-formulated as the CDT. According to the CDT the underlying cause of dyslexia is a cerebellar impairment. Cerebellar dysfunction has been linked to a range of behavioural deficits, such as problems in: 1) motor skills (Holmes, 1939), 2) automatisation of motor skills (Ito, 1990), 3) classical conditioning of the eyeblink response (Daum et al., 1993) and 4) perception and production of timing tasks (Ivry and Keele, 1989).

Research on dyslexia by Nicolson and Fawcet reported that DPs indeed have deficits over a range of functions which rely on cerebellar processing, such as: motor skills, including balancing – a gross motor skill, (Fawcett and Nicolson, 1999), eye-blink conditioning (Nicolson, Daum, Schugens, Fawcett, and Schulz, 2002) and time estimation (Nicolson et al., 1995). Note, however, that a recent meta-analysis (Rochelle and Talcott, 2006) showed that balance deficit in dyslexia can be accounted for by comorbid developmental disorders, such as ADHD and DCD (see also Wimmer, Mayringer, and Raberger, 1999). For further details on the CDT please see reviews (Fawcett and Nicolson, 2004; Nicolson and Fawcett, 2008; Nicolson et al., 2001).

On the basis of findings implicating cerebellar impairment in dyslexia, Nicolson et al. (2001) proposed a hypothetical ontogenetic causal chain linking cerebellar impairment with phonological and reading deficits, (as well as with spelling and hand writing deficits). According to this model there are two routes by which cerebellar impairment could lead to reading difficulties in dyslexia. According to the first - a major route, cerebellar impairment (probably dating back to gestation) leads to mild articulatory problems, which lead to an impoverished representation of the phonological characteristics of speech. This in turn leads to difficulties in phonological awareness at approximately five years of age and subsequently results in difficulties with learning to read. Additionally, reduced articulation speed leads to reduced working memory.

According to the second route, difficulties in reading acquisition stem from cerebellar impairment which causes problems with automatizing skills and knowledge, leading to difficulties with: 1) automatic grapheme-phoneme conversion, 2) automatic word recognition, 3) automatic verbal working memory and 4) automatic awareness of the orthographic regularities of a given language.

According to this hypothetical ontogenetic causal chain, cerebellar impairment is also the underlying cause of impairment of motor skills which leads to writing impairment (dysgraphia). Furthermore, cerebellar deficit leads to balance deficits. However, it is not these motor difficulties (with the exception of the articulatory motor difficulties) and problems with balance that leads to reading difficulties (Nicolson et al., 2001) but the underlying cerebellar deficit.

1.5. Neuroimaging Studies (Mainly Involving Tasks Specifically Developed to Probe Phonological, Visual Magnocellular and Cerebellar Function) Which Have a Bearing on the Main Theories of Dyslexia

There have been a number of neuroimaging studies - some with CPs and some comparing DPs and CPs, with the latter motivated by each of the three current main theories of dyslexia, but conducted with the focus usually on one theoretical framework. The results from these studies have a bearing on the PDT, visual MDT and CDT.

Before reviewing the neuroimaging studies three issues need to be introduced: 1) labelling conventions of brain areas; 2) brain activation and 3) the related terms of *overactivation* and *underactivation*. Regarding the first, there are a number of different ways to label a given brain area. One of the oldest systems, which is still widely used is a system invented by Korbinian Brodmann who reported the cytoarchitectural organization of neurons in the cerebral cortex using the Nissl stain. Each area was given a unique number and labelled, for instance BA44, where ‘BA’ stands for Brodmann area and 44 is the unique number. Nowadays Brodmann’s areas are in common use for descriptive purposes (Crossman and Neary, 2005). Although Brodmann’s map and cytoarchitectonic analysis constitute a considerable scientific achievement, recent data obtained using imaging techniques underscore several shortcomings of these early architectonic maps. These include: 1) their presentation in two-dimensional schematic drawings; 2) the definition of the criteria which describe a given cortical area and its borders are observer dependent; and 3) the fact that inter-participant differences in brain architecture and macroscopy were neglected. These criticisms have been addressed in the seminal work of Karl Zilles and his colleagues (Zilles, Schleicher, Palomero-Gallagher, and Amunts, 2002) and incorporated, in this chapter. All areas investigated in this chapter, for which there are probabilistic cytoarchitectonic labels, were labeled as such, using the Anatomy Toolbox V.1.8 (AT) (Eickhoff et al., 2005) (please see section ‘ROI analysis (mask)’ for more details). Two areas (the L middle temporal gyrus and L fusiform gyrus) for which there are no probabilistic cytoarchitectonic labels, were labelled using macroanatomically defined brain regions (Tzourio-Mazoyer et al., 2002). Areas reported from studies by other authors are always reported using the same labels as in the original source.

With regard to the issue of brain activation - it is measured in fMRI experiments by the BOLD (Blood Oxygenation Level Dependent) contrast (Matthews, 2001; Ugurbil, 2002). The terms ‘activates’, ‘activated’, ‘activation’ refer to localised changes in BOLD which: 1) do not provide a direct measure of neuronal activity and 2) are related to the neural activity evoked by a given experimental task, such as, deciding whether a given pair of consonants rhyme. ‘Activation’ is usually relative to a control condition, such as deciding whether a Korean letter looks similar to a Korean target letter (Paulesu et al., 1996).

The third issue has to do with two terms related to the term ‘activation’. *Underactivation* (synonymous with the term *hypoactivation*) – can be defined as activation which is significantly less than a given activation. *Overactivation* (synonymous term – *hyperactivation*) can be defined as activation which is significantly greater than a given activation. It is common to observe underactivation and overactivation in the neuroimaging studies of patients as compared to the control group (Hoeft et al., 2007), of DPs in comparison with the CPs (Hoeft et al., 2007) and in neuroimaging studies of normal aging in older participants, as compared to younger participants (Cabeza, Anderson, Locantore, and McIntosh, 2002).

1.5.1. Neuroimaging Studies Testing the Phonological Skills of CPs

The deficit postulated by the PDT has also been specified on the biological level as the L Perisylvian region abnormality (Frith, 1997) or more recently as the L temporo-parietal abnormality and L frontal abnormality (Hulme and Snowling, 2009). As these descriptive terms seem not to be detailed enough to thoroughly test the PDT on the neural level, the approach taken in this chapter is as follows.First the neuroimaging studies, which have tested the involvement of brain areas used in phonological processing, are reviewed below. The studies, to be included, had to investigate phonological processing using classical tests which tap into phonological processing, namely: *phonological awareness*, *naming* and *short term memory* tasks. The other criterion here was that the studies had to focus either on just CPs, or on DPs (as compared with the CPs). Second, the areas which consistently come up in these studies, as involved in phonological processing, were used in this study to test the PDT. The role of these areas was also validated with the broader literature review presented in the section 'Brain regions and associated phonological processing' which follows the review of the neuroimaging studies on phonological awareness, naming and short term memory, included below.

Neuroimaging studies on CPs have shown that *phonological awareness* tasks which involve segmented phonology (e.g. silently making a decision whether a given consonant rhymes with another consonant – "Does *'p'* rhyme with *'t'* ?") activate the perisylvian structures in the L (left) hemisphere, including: the L inferior frontal gyrus - BA44/45 (Broca's area), the L posterior superior temporal gyrus - BA22/21 (including Wernicke's area), the L insula, as well as the L SMA (supplementary motor area) (BA6) and L PMC premotor cortex (BA6) (Paulesu et al., 1996) (some other areas were also activated please see Appendix A, Table 1).

Phonological awareness studies which involved word rhyming in CPs (e.g., Booth, Wood, Lu, Houk, and Bitan, 2007; Xu et al., 2001) also revealed activation in Broca's and Wernicke's areas, however, additionally the L fusiform gyrus (BA19/37) and L inferior temporal occipital junction (BA37) were activated. Nonword rhyming, similarly to word rhyming, activated the L inferior temporal occipital junction (BA37) in CPs, but additionally the L supramarginal gyrus (BA40) was activated (Xu et al., 2001) (for details, including other activated areas, please see Appendix A, Table 1).

Neuroimaging studies of *covert object naming* (a task where a participant is asked to fixate on the visually presented object and to think silently of its name) (single item per trial) elicited activation in Broca's and Wernicke's areas, the L posterior fusiform gyrus (BA37), L middle temporal gyrus (BA21) and L premotor cortex (Lurito et al., 2000; Moore and Price, 1999). Other areas were also involved (please see Appendix A, Table 1).

Moving on to investigations of *verbal short term memory* in CPs, Paulesu et al. (1996) conducted a study where participants were instructed to remember sequences of six consonants and, two seconds later, to make a judgement whether a target consonant appeared in the previously presented sequence. CPs exhibited a similar pattern of activations to those evoked in the consonant rhyming task reported above (Paulesu et al., 1996). The following areas were activated: the L inferior frontal gyrus (BA6/44), SMA (BA6), PMC (BA6), the L insula, L superior temporal gyrus (BA22) and the L supramarginal gyrus (BA40). Other areas were also activated (please see Appendix A, Table 1). Moreover, a study by Paulesu, Frith, and Frackowiak (1993) confirmed the crucial role of the supramarginal gyrus (BA 40) in verbal short term memory.

1.5.2. Neuroimaging Studies Testing the Phonological Skills of DPs (As Compared to CPs)

Investigations of phonological processing in DPs, similar to the studies on CPs, have included *phonological awareness, naming* and *short-term memory* tasks. The aforementioned study by Paulesu et al. (1996) also investigated the performance of DPs in a covert consonant rhyming task. The results revealed that DPs exhibited significantly less activation than CPs in the L superior temporal gyrus (BA21/22), L insula and the L premotor cortex (PMC) (BA6). Some other areas were also involved (please see Appendix A, Table 1).

A further study by Shaywitz et al. (1998) with a sample of teenage and adult DPs, used (among others) the *covert single letter rhyming* task. This is a task where the subject views two simultaneously presented stimuli, e.g., [*t*] and [*v*], one above the other, and is asked to indicate (by pressing an appropriate response button) whether these letters rhyme. The authors found that DPs exhibited significantly less activation in L posterior areas: the angular gyrus (BA39) and the posterior superior temporal gyrus (BA22). The other areas significantly less activated by DPs involved the striate cortex (BA17) and the R hemisphere homologues. In contrast, when performing the same task DPs showed significantly more activation than CPs in the L inferior frontal gyrus, including the pars opercularis (BA44) and pars triangularis (BA45) and their R hemisphere homologues (R BA44 and R BA45). Shaywitz et al. (1998) concluded that the results support the PDT.

Regarding *naming* in DPs and CPs, McCrory, Mechelli, Frith and Price (2005) used a PET study to look for a common neurological impairment for reading and naming deficit in DPs. The results revealed that despite their unimpaired behavioural performance, DPs showed significantly less activation during picture naming and reading words in the L occipito-temporal area. Interestingly, the reduced activation for these tasks in DPs corresponds to 'the visual word form area' (VWFA) – claimed by some researchers (Cohen et al., 2000; Cohen et al., 2002; Cohen et al., 2003) to be specific to orthographic processing. McCrory et al. (2005), on the basis of their results demonstrating activation in both reading and picture naming (which does not involve orthographic processing), concluded that the L occipito-temporal area cannot be specific to orthographic processing, as claimed earlier (Cohen et al., 2000; Cohen et al., 2002; Cohen et al., 2003), but must be involved in a more general deficit in binding visual with phonological information (for further discussion see Cohen and Dehaene, 2004; Price and Devlin, 2003).

Finally, Paulesu et al.'s (1996) study, described above, also investigated *verbal short term memory* which taps into phonological processing in DPs and CPs. CPs exhibited a similar pattern of activation to that found in other neuroimaging studies of short term memory (e.g., Paulesu et al., 1993). The largest differences between DPs and CPs were noted in Broca's area (BA44) and in the L insula. In contrast, no significant differences between the groups in this task were found in Wernicke's area. The other areas where DPs exhibited significantly less activation included: the L SMA (BA6) and L superior middle gyrus (BA40) (for further details and other areas involved, please see Appendix A, Table 1). On the basis of the neuroimaging results from this experiment and the consonant rhyming experiment reported above, the authors put forward a hypothesis that dyslexia may be caused by a disconnection between the anterior and posterior language areas. The authors proposed that this could be due to an impaired L insula which may act as an anatomical bridge between Broca's area and the superior temporal cortex, and inferior parietal cortex. This interpretation, taken together with other findings, suggests that there may be different types of phonological deficit, some to do with disconnection between the involved areas and some with deficit within the involved areas.

It is important to point out here that the update of the PDT (Hulme and Snowling, 2009) postulates that abnormality in the L anterior areas (together with abnormality in the L temporo-parietal areas) are the underlying cause of reading impairment in dyslexia. The earlier version of the PDT (Frith, 1997) did not include the anterior areas. As the L frontal anterior areas are involved in phonological processing (please see details below), it is only natural (from the perspective of the PDT) to assume that they could be the underlying cause of reading impairment. However, the literature reviewed (see the section 'Neuroimaging studies of reading in adult DPs, as compared to CPs' below) shows that the anterior areas are overactivated in some studies and this overactivation has been interpreted as a manifestation of a compensatory mechanism.

As a range of areas was activated in the phonological tasks, as discussed above, it is not clear whether they are all necessary for phonological processing. The role of the areas, which have also been validated as involved in phonological processing by other studies, is discussed below in more detail. These areas are then used in the study presented in this chapter for testing the PDT.

1.5.3. Brain Regions and Associated Phonological Processing

In 1861, Paul Broca reported a postmortem study of a patient who suffered from language articulation impairment. The results revealed that the patient had damage in the L hemisphere third frontal convolution. By deduction, Paul Broca associated this area with the motor images of speech. The involvement of Broca's area (BA44/45) in phonological processing has been consistently underscored (e.g., Gainotti, Miceli, Silveri, and Villa, 1982). Current neuroimaging evidence suggests that Broca's area seems to play a major role in the phonological rehearsal system (Paulesu et al., 1996). It also plays a role in segmented phonology, which involves representations of the separated sub-syllabic components, such as onsets and 'rimes', e.g., *'b'* and *'ee'*, in case of the item *'bee'* (Paulesu et al., 1996). BA44 has been hypothesised to be involved in: sub-vocal rehearsal (Paulesu et al., 1996), short term memory (Romero, Walsh, and Papagno, 2006), support of grapheme-to-phoneme conversion (Heim et al., 2005) and performance of sensory-motor integration during sublexical processing (on the level of sublexical units, such as phonemes) (Hickok and Poeppel, 2004). BA45 has been associated with explicit lexical search (Heim et al., 2005).

In 1874 Carl Wernicke reported a postmortem study of a patient who had problems with speech comprehension. The results showed that the patient had damage in the L hemisphere posterior superior temporal cortex (known nowadays as Wernicke's area). Carl Wernicke associated this area with the auditory images of speech. Since then the role of Wernicke's area (BA22) has been consistently implicated in phonological processing (e.g., Seines, Knopman, Niccum, and Rubens, 1985). This area is hypothesised to be involved in the processing of unsegmented phonology (e.g., phoneme *'[b]'*). As Wernicke's area is also activated by language tasks which do not involve auditory language input (Price, Wise, and Frackowiak, 1996) some authors (Paulesu et al., 1996) have proposed that Wernicke's area may be involved in phonological modality-independent representations.

The L middle temporal gyrus (BA21) is argued to be the substrate for lexical representation (Poeppel, Idsardi, and Wassenhove, 2009). It is activated in neuroimaging studies which tap into phonological and semantic processing (Lurito et al., 2000; McDermott,

Petersen, Watson, and Ojemann, 2003; Moore and Price, 1999; Tivarus, Hillier, Schmalbrock, and Beversdorf, 2008). It is also involved in speech comprehension at the sentence level (Price, 2010).

Although the insula has long been implicated in phonological processing (e.g., Damasio and Damasio, 1980), its role was not clear. Paulesu et al. (1996) hypothesised that the role of the L insula is to convert unsegmented and segmented phonological codes between Broca's area, the superior temporal cortex and the inferior parietal cortex.

Damage to the L supramarginal gyrus (part of the L inferior parietal lobule; part of BA40) (together with damage to BA39, please see below) was described as early as 1891 by Dejerine (1891, 1892; cited in Shaywitz et al., 2001). Dejerine suggested that the L supramarginal gyrus (with angular gyrus) is critical for reading. The role of the L supramarginal gyrus in phonological processing was implicated in studies on patient populations (e.g., Benson et al., 1973; Kertesz, Harlock, and Coates, 1979; Warrington, Logue, and Pratt, 1971). The results of neuroimaging studies have suggested that the L supramarginal gyrus may act as a 'phonological storehouse' that becomes activated for word retrieval (Paulesu et al., 1993; Paulesu et al., 1996; Price, Moore, Humphreys, and Wise, 1997). More recently, it has been suggested (Zatorre and Gandour, 2009) that this area supports phonological encoding-recoding processes in a variety of different tasks. It is engaged in phonological short-term memory (Paulesu et al., 1993; Romero et al., 2006). Furthermore, it also supports both phonological and semantic processing in reading (Stoeckel, Gough, Watkins, and Devlin, 2009).

Damage to L angular gyrus (BA39; situated in the L inferior parietal lobule) was described by Dejerine (1891, 1892; cited in Price, 2000) in patients who had alexia with agraphia. Hence, the L angular gyrus has been historically linked to memories of visual word forms. More recently the L angular gyrus started to be considered as a part of an association cortex which is involved in cross-modal mapping of graphemes to phonemes (Geschwind, 1965; Shaywitz et al., 1998). (There is also evidence that the L angular gyrus plays a role in semantic processing (Price, 2000)).

The anterior aspect of the L precentral gyrus PMC (Premotor cortex) (BA6), also known as SMA (the supplementary motor area) is involved in both vocalisation of speech and sub-vocalisation of speech (internal speech). It is activated both for reading aloud and silently (Dietz, Jones, Gareau, Zeffiro, and Eden, 2005) and is associated with the initiation of speech. It was reported (Mesulam, 1990) that lesions of this area result in transcortical motor aphasia.

The L fusiform gyrus (BA 19/37) is engaged in word rhyming tasks (relative to visual baseline) (Booth et al., 2007) and covert object naming (Lurito et al., 2000; Moore and Price, 1999). It was reported (Brockway, 2011) that electrical stimulation of the fusiform gyrus, with grid electrodes, during computerised speech and object naming tasks, resulted in language deficits including speech arrest, dysnomia and jargon aphasia.

Finally, according to McCrory et al. (2005) the L posterior fusiform gyrus (also known as VWFA) is involved in a general deficit in binding visual with phonological information. Its function is most likely not limited to reading, but it is also engaged when processing any meaningful visual stimulus (Devlin, Jamison, Gonnerman, and Matthews, 2006) (for further discussion see Cohen and Dehaene, 2004; Price and Devlin, 2003).

Summarising, although it is not currently clear which areas are crucial for phonological processing, the areas described above seem to be good candidates for testing the PDT and are therefore used for this purpose in this chapter.

1.5.4. Neuroimaging Studies Investigating Visual Magnocellular Processing

With regard to the visual MDT (which claims that the underlying cause of literacy problems in dyslexia is a more general impairment of the visual magnocellular system with spared parvocellular system), motion perception is widely used to tap into magnocellular processing (Cornelissen, Richardson, Mason, Fowler, and Stein, 1995; Newsome and Pare, 1988; Samar and Parasnis, 2005; Stein, 2001). Human homologues of motion sensitive areas, which were originally identified in monkey's brain, have been reported, e.g., V5/MT (Zeki et al., 1991), V3a (Tootell et al., 1997) and V6/V6a (Dechent and Frahm, 2003). Interestingly, V1 (striate cortex) and V2 (extrastriate cortex) areas were active not only for colour, but also for motion stimulation (Zeki et al., 1991), confirming that V1 and V2 are characterised by magnocellular input, as well as parvocellular input.

Moving on to the neuroimaging studies which have a bearing on the visual MDT in the context of reading, a study by Liederman et al. (2003) is of importance. The study investigated: 1) a task which biased towards phonological processing (participants had to indicate whether pronounceable non-word letter strings sounded like real English words) and 2) non-word reading. During these tasks, in unimpaired adults, the processing in V5/MT+ was disrupted using rTMS (repeated Transcranial Magnetic Stimulation - a neurophysiological technique which can be used to induce an electric current in the brain using a magnetic field which crosses the scull, disrupting sensory and cognitive processing by creating temporary 'virtual lesions' (Pascual-Leone and Walsh, 2002)). The results revealed that there was no effect of rTMS on a task which biased towards phonological processing. This suggests that the grapheme to phoneme transformation process was intact after rTMS was applied to V5/MT+. On the basis of this result the authors concluded that the process by which V5/MT+ is correlated with rate of reading is not likely to be due to a direct role of V5/MT+ in phonological processing. In contrast, the results revealed significantly decreased performance on non-word reading, compared to the condition where no rTMS stimulation was applied. Error analysis showed that most errors involved vowels and consonants and consisted of substitutions, omissions, position changes and additions. Phonological errors, in nonword reading defined as: changes in voicing, in place of articulation, in manner of articulation, cases of labialisation, gliding, depalatelisation or stopping almost never occurred.

The significance of Liederman et al.'s (2003) findings is that they demonstrated that V5/ MT+ (traditionally labelled as a 'visual motion area') is also implicated in the reading process, not by being directly involved in phonological processing, but most likely by image stabilisation and/or letter localisation. This role of V5/MT+ was inferred on the basis of the visual errors which occurred in non-word reading during virtual lesions of V5/MT+. This finding suggests that the processing in V5/MT+ has an independent contribution to the reading process from that of the areas responsible for phonological processing. Importantly, this aspect of magnocellular involvement in the reading process should be relevant throughout most of the life-span of a given individual – usually from reading acquisition age to death.

Regarding findings on DPs, four studies need to be mentioned here (Demb, Boynton, and Heeger, 1997; 1998; Eden et al., 1996; Vanni, Uusitalo, Kiesila, and Hari, 1997). Eden et al. (1996) showed, in an fMRI study, that the presentation of moving stimuli in a motion coherence task failed to detect activation in V5/MT in DPs, as compared to CPs (please see Appendix A, Table 2). Conversely, presentation of visual stationary patterns, in the control condition, elicited equivalent activations in V1/V2 and the extrastriate cortex in DPs and CPs.

These results were obtained in both the single participant analysis and the between-group analysis.

In two other fMRI studies, which investigated magnocellular processing (Demb et al., 1997; 1998), the authors found that DPs showed significantly lower responses than CPs in V5/MT+ (and other extrastriate areas, including: V1, V2, V3, V3a and V4v) when responding to moving visual grating stimuli presented at a low mean luminance. Such stimuli, likely stimulate magnocellular inputs to cortex (Purpura, Kaplan, and Shapley, 1988). On the other hand, DPs were not impaired when responding in the control condition to contrast-reversing grating stimuli presented at a higher mean luminance. There were significant correlations (assessed jointly for DPs and CPs) between brain activity under low mean luminance moving grating conditions and reading rate in all investigated areas. There was a range of contrasts for which the correlations were significant, including: V5/MT+ (3 to 100%), V1 (31 to 100%), V2 (54 to 100%), V3 (52 to 100%), V3A (14 to 92%) and V4v (70 to 100%). The authors interpreted their findings as being consistent with a specific magnocellular pathway deficit in dyslexia.

Although Demb et al. (1997; 1998) demonstrated significant differences between DPs and CPs, the authors, in contrast to Eden et al.'s (1996) study, found activation of V5/MT+ in DPs in response to moving versus stationary dot patterns. Furthermore, the results involving V1/V2 (Demb et al., 1997; 1998) are not consistent with Eden et al.'s (1996) study. Different results for V5/MT+ and V1/V2 in these two studies could be due to the different samples of DPs or to different magnocellular tasks. However, Demb et al. (1997; 1998) advocate that their results provide support for a magnocellular pathway deficit in dyslexia. The main finding comes from the significant differences between DPs and CPs in V5/MT+ activity for stimuli which elicit activity from magnocellular inputs to the brain as early as V1.

Vanni, Uusitalo, Kiesila, and Hari (1997), on the other hand, reported a study that used magnetoencephalography (MEG) (a non-invasive neuroimaging technique which directly records weak magnetic fields generated by electrical currents in the brain (Hämäläinen and Hari, 2002)). Both high and low contrast motion stimuli elicited similar activation in DPs and CPs in V5/MT. This result is not consistent with the M-pathway deficit which would predict impairment at low contrast motion stimuli, but not at high contrast motion stimuli. The finding that the authors were able to localise V5/MT in DPs is in line with Demb et al.'s (1997; 1998), but not with Eden et al.'s (1996) findings. The result of not finding significant differences in activation patterns between the CPs and DPs in V5/MT contrasts with Demb et al.'s (1997; 1998) and Eden et al.'s (1996) results. It is not clear what underlies this difference, it may be because of different samples of DPs, different experimental stimuli, or different techniques used, with MEG, in contrast to fMRI, being able to pick up small and transient changes in neuronal oscillatory power. The different samples of DPs is a likely source of the discrepant results, because there is high heterogeneity among DPs some of whom exhibit a magnocellular deficit and some of whom do not (Ramus et al., 2003; Reid et al., 2007).

1.5.5. Neuroimaging Studies Investigating the Cerebellum

The role of the cerebellum has traditionally been associated with balance, posture, muscle tone, walking, coordination of movement in precise motor tasks (such as performing surgery), visual guidance of movement and the motor aspects of articulation (Brodal, 1981; Fiez and Raichle, 1997; Holmes, 1939; Kiernan, 2009; Snell, 2001; Stein and Glickstein, 1992).

However, since approximately 20 years ago (with improved technology to image the whole brain) there is now growing evidence that the cerebellum is involved in cognitive tasks, including language (for reviews see Fiez and Raichle, 1997; Marien, Engelborghs, Fabbro, and De Deyn, 2001; Schmahmann, 1997; Stoodley, 2012; Stoodley and Schmahmann, 2009; Stoodley, Valera, and Schmahmann, 2012). However, involvement of the cerebellum in cognitive tasks has met with considerable controversy (for a comprehensive summary of older and modern approaches to studying and understanding the role of the cerebellum, see Manto, Gruol, Schmahmann, Koibuchi, and Rossi, 2013; Schmahmann, 1997).

Leiner, Leiner and Dow (1993) reported that the human cerebellum, especially the cerebellar ventro-lateral dentate nucleus and lateral cerebellar hemispheres, evolved in humans to become connected not only with the frontal lobe motor areas, but also with Broca's area, incorporating the cerebellum into the language network.

Regarding neuroimaging studies with CPs, which have a bearing on the CDT, an fMRI study (Fulbright et al., 1999) which investigated cerebellar activation during reading with adult CPs, needs to be mentioned here (for more details on studies involving the cerebellum please see Appendix A, Table 3). It investigated, among other conditions, two tasks: a rhyming judgement for pseudoword pairs (e.g., Does *leat* rhyme with *jete*?) and a semantic category judgement for real words (Do *man* and *boy* belong to the same semantic category?), both relative to a control task requiring judgements of line orientation. The results revealed differential patterns of activation in the cerebellum between these two tasks. In the first task, which heavily relied on phonological processing, cerebellar activation was noted in the middle and posterior aspects of the posterior superior fissure and adjacent (bilateral) hemispheric (H) simple lobule (R and L H lobule VI) and semilunar lobule bilaterally. Activation was also found in posterior aspects of the simple lobule, superior semilunar lobule (R and L H Crus I), and inferior semilunar lobule (R and L H Crus II, and R and L H lobule VIIB). In contrast, the second task, which largely relies on semantic processing, elicited activation in the deep nuclear region on the right and in the inferior vermis, in addition to the posterior areas activated in the phonological task reported above. The significance of this study lies in the fact that it clearly shows that the cerebellum, among other areas, plays a role in phonological and semantic processing during reading. Furthermore, a recent meta-analysis (Stoodley and Schmahmann, 2009) of fMRI studies confirmed that the cerebellum subserves language processing; this conclusion is based on the broad range of language processing studies in this meta-analysis, including: word generation, phonological, semantic and morphological processing. The areas with significant activation likelihood estimate included: R H lobule VI, R H Crus I, R H Crus I/II, R Vermal lobule VIIAt, L H lobule VI and L H Crus I. Note that L H Crus I was not reported in Stoodley and Schmahmann' s (2009) publication, however, the MNI coordinates (x=-42, y=-58, z=-26) given in this publication were labelled with the AT as L H Crus I (and as L Lobule VI (Hem) (please see Table 1).

As stated earlier, according to the CDT (Nicolson et al., 2001) the underlying cause of dyslexia is a cerebellar impairment. The exact nature of the cerebellar deficit is not specified, hence studies have probed the whole range of cerebellar function in DPs, as compared to CPs. The support for this theory came first from behavioural studies which tested cerebellar function, such as eye-blink conditioning (Nicolson, Daum, Schugens, Fawcett, and Schulz, 2002). However, more recently a significant number of neuroimaging studies (using various neuroimaging techniques) have reported evidence that there are significant differences between DPs and CPs in the cerebellum. These neuroimaging studies are reviewed below.

Brain activation was shown to be significantly lower in adult DPs compared to CPs in the R cerebellar cortex when learning a new sequence of finger presses and in the R cerebellar cortex (and the L cingulate gyrus) when performing a pre-learned sequence of finger presses (Nicolson et al., 1999).

A more recent fMRI study with child DPs (Baillieux et al., 2009) used a noun-verb association paradigm where high frequency nouns were presented via headphones and participants had to silently generate a semantically related verb. The results showed that CPs, in comparison to DPs, exhibited activation in the anterior and posterior areas of the cerebellar hemispheres (R lobule V, R and L lobule VI and L lobule VIIIA). In contrast, DPs showed activation only in the posterior areas of the cerebellar hemispheres (L lobule VI, L Curs I and R Crus II). However, DPs also showed activation in the anterior and posterior parts of the Vermis (R lobule I and II, R lobule III, L lobule V and R lobule VIIAt and VIIAf). These results suggest that the pattern of activation in the cerebellum in DPs (as compared with CPs) is atypical during language processing. One must be cautious, however, when making a comparison with the results reported by Baillieux et al. (2009) because due to small sample size, the results are based on a fixed effect analysis which does not allow generalisation onto the population of DPs and they also refer only to child DPs.

Converging evidence for anatomical cerebellar abnormalities in dyslexia has come from studies based on neuroimaging methods other than fMRI, including magnetic resonance spectroscopy and histological studies. Rae et al. (1998), used magnetic resonance spectroscopy (MRS) (a technique which uses magnetic resonance imaging to detect concentrations of low-molecular-weight metabolites *in vivo* (Maudsley, 2002)), and found significant differences in concentrations of some neurometabolites in the cerebellum of adult DPs as compared to CPs. The study revealed that the Cho/Na ratio (choline-containing compounds/N-acetylaspartate) was significantly lower in DPs than in CPs in particular brain areas, most likely due to a decrease of Cho and increase of Na in DPs. As 'Cho' is believed to be a surrogate marker of overall cellular density and 'Na' is a surrogate marker of neuronal density, the authors interpreted these differences as resulting from a decrease in total cell membranes, without a corresponding decrease in the total neuronal volume. A more recent study (Laycock et al., 2008), also using spectroscopy, found that DPs exhibited a higher ratio of Cho/Cr (creatine) in the L cerebellar hemisphere accompanied by a lower ratio of Na/Cho in the R cerebellar hemisphere. Furthermore, cerebellar white and grey matter volumes of the same DPs and CPs were investigated using volumetric MRI. The results revealed that DPs had a larger volume of white matter in L and R cerebellar hemispheres than CPs. The authors stated that both results could be accounted for by abnormal myelination or excessive connectivity in the cerebellum of DPs.

Further evidence on cerebellar abnormalities in DPs comes from studies using structural MRI. Structural MRI is often analysed using voxel-based morphometry (VBM), a technique, which in its simplest form, investigates a voxel-wise comparison of the local concentration of grey matter between two groups of participants (Ashburner and Friston, 2000). In contrast to traditional morphometry, which involves measuring the volume of the whole brain or its subparts, risking that smaller differences in volume may be overlooked, in VBM the image volume is compared across brains at every voxel. Significantly smaller grey matter volume in DPs than CPs has been reported in the following cerebellar areas: the bilateral anterior cerebellum (Kronbichler et al., 2008), the L semilunar lobule (Brown et al., 2001; Eckert et al., 2003) and R semilunar lobule (Brown et al., 2001).

It has also been reported (Rae et al., 2002) that DPs, exhibited grey matter symmetry of the L and R cerebellum. This contrasted with the findings for CPs who showed significantly more grey matter in the R cerebellum than in the L cerebellum. DPs' degree of cerebellar symmetry was correlated with the severity of their phonological decoding deficit. Moreover, Pernet, Poline, Demonet, and Rousselet (2009), used CPs' brains to build a 'typical' brain using bootstrapped confidence intervals. Pernet et al. (2009) repeated the sampling 4999 times (a total of 5000 samples). The authors obtained a distribution of bootstrapped estimates of the mean, averaged across subjects. The 95% percent confidence intervals were calculated based on the histograms (alpha=0.05)). Each DP's grey matter was classified at each voxel as being outside or within the normal range, as determined by CPs. The results revealed that the grey matter volume of the R cerebellar declive (R Vermal lobule VI) (and the R lentiform nucleus) differentiated DPs and CPs in such a way that 100% of DPs fell outside the 95% confidence interval boundaries of CPs. DPs with lower cerebellar declive grey matter volumes performed worse than participants with higher cerebellar declive grey matter volumes in phonological tasks.

Finally, evidence on cerebellar abnormalities comes from a post-mortem histological study of the cerebellum by Finch, Nicolson, and Fawcett (2002). The authors investigated the size and density of cerebellar Purkinje cells (some of the largest (GABAergic) neurons in the human brain, found only in the cerebellum), with samples systematically taken from the anterior, posterior and flocculonodular lobes. Finch et al. (2002) used the same specimens from the Orton Society brain bank, as Galaburda and colleagues used, to determine abnormalities in the magnocellular layers of the LGN in DPs' brains (e.g., Galaburda and Kemper, 1979; Galaburda, Sherman, Rosen, Aboitiz, and Geschwind, 1985). The cell size analysis revealed that Purkinje cells were significantly larger in DPs than in CPs in the posterior cerebellar cortex. No significant differences between the groups were found in the anterior and flocculonodular lobes. Distributional analyses showed significant differences in posterior and anterior lobes due to DPs having more large Purkinje cells and fewer small Purkinje cells. Currently it is not clear what effect these differences in cell sizes may have; one possible difference on the neuropsychological level would perhaps be increased oxygen utilisation in DPs with more large Purkinje cells. The biggest difference between the groups was noted in the medial Crus II and paramedian lobule (VIIB). Both these areas receive somatotopic information. For instance, the paramedian lobule (VIIB) exhibited a rise to action potentials during stimulation (natural or electrical) from skin or cutaneous nerves. The paramedian lobule (VIIB) has a representation of the whole body (Brodal, 1981), while the medial Crus II receives input from the peri-oral and intra-oral structures. This result suggests differences in DPs, as compared to CPs, in the representation of head or upper body. The authors interpreted the finding as being consistent with Fawcett, Nicolson, and Dean's (1996) hypothesis according to which cerebellar deficit may cause early speech problems because fluent speech requires coordination of articulators in the neck and head. Furthermore, there were no significant differences between DPs and CPs in the dentate nucleus. In contrast, the groups differed in the distribution of Purkinje cell sizes in the inferior olive, due to fewer small Purkinje cells and more large Purkinje cells in DPs than in CPs.

According to Finch et al. (2002), the abnormality patterns, found in the histological study described above, are in line with the hypothesis that the problems in dyslexia are to do with the input side (especially the error feedback loop which is mediated in the inferior olive by the climbing fibres) and not with the hypothesis that the deficits are to do with the output side to the dentate nucleus (Nicolson and Fawcett, 2008). For clarity, the input and output cerebellar pathways, as well as a model of the cerebellar error feedback loop, are briefly described below.

It has been postulated that the cerebellar cortex contains relatively independent microzones which consist of Purkinje cells and their associated inputs and outputs (Ito, 2000). In combination with associated pathways from and to deep cerebellar nuclei, a given microzone may be conceptualised as a microcomplex which can undertake different tasks. The Purkinje cells receive input from: 1) up to 175,000 parallel fibres formed from the granule cells' axons and 2) one climbing fibre from the inferior olivary nucleus which makes up to 20,000 synapses with the Purkinje cell. The cortico-olivary fibres arise from neurons in the temporal, parietal, frontal and occipital lobes, go through the corona radiata and internal capsule and terminate in the L and R inferior olivary nuclei. Fibres from the inferior olivary nuclei cross the middle and enter the contralateral cerebellar hemisphere. These fibres terminate as the climbing fibres in the cerebellum. This pathway is known as the cerebro-olivocerebellar pathway (Snell, 2001) which is afferent and therefore concerned with input.

The dentate nucleus is one of the deep cerebellar nuclei. Axons of neurons in this nucleus go through the superior cerebellar peduncle and cross the middle to the contralateral side. The fibres end by synapsing with cells in the ventrolateral nucleus of the contralateral thalamus. The axons of thalamic neurons go through the internal capsule and corona radiata and terminate in the cerebral cortex. This is known as the dento-thalamic pathway (Snell, 2001) and it is efferent in nature, hence concerned with the output.

Many different models of cerebellar function have been hypothesised, however the Marr/Albus composite model is still currently valid for skill execution and acquisition (Ito, 2000). The Marr/Albus model hypothesises that the climbing fibres act as an error signal to the cerebellar microzone, constituting an inner loop.

Summarising, a considerable number of neuroimaging studies (using various neuroimaging techniques) have reported significant differences between DPs and CPs in the cerebellum. These findings provide some support for the CDT. If the underlying cause of dyslexia is a cerebellar deficit, as claimed by the CDT, then the cerebellum should be a good candidate to consider when trying to establish the neural correlates of reading impairment in dyslexia.

1.5.6. Summary of the Neuroimaging Studies Motivated by the Main Theories of Dyslexia, Criticisms and the Approach Taken in the Research Presented in This Chapter

In summary, neuroimaging studies based on samples from the non-reading impaired population provide potentially important insights into the neural correlates of phonological, visual magnocellular and cerebellar processing. Guided by these frameworks, studies comparing DPs with CPs have revealed some support for the existence of phonological, visual magnocellular and cerebellar deficits in dyslexia. With few exceptions (e.g., Eden et al., 1996), these neuroimaging studies, have involved only group comparisons. Given that recent research on dyslexia emphasises the heterogeneity of the deficits in this developmental disorder (Heim et al., 2008; Menghini et al., 2010; Ramus et al., 2003; Reid et al., 2007; Snowling, 2008), it is unclear what proportion of DPs exhibit a specific functional and/or structural brain abnormality consistent with each of these causal theories.

Currently it is not clear why there are so many heterogeneous deficits in dyslexia. As described at the beginning of this chapter, definitions of dyslexia state that this disorder mainly affects literacy (i.e. reading impairment) (American Psychiatric Association, 1994; British Dyslexia Association, 2007; International Dyslexia Association, 2009; World Federation of Neurology, 1968). Therefore to uncover the core neural correlates of impairment in developmental dyslexia, one needs to uncover the neural correlates of a reading disorder (which occurs in dyslexia, despite normal IQ, normal cognitive skills, appropriate motivation and education, and lack of any known cognitive and psychiatric disorders). However, the majority of neuroimaging studies, motivated by the main theories of dyslexia have focused on hypothesised deficits in DPs without demonstrating a relationship with reading disorder. Demonstration of a significant between group (DPs and CPs) difference on a given variable (e.g., time estimation measurement) does not necessarily demonstrate a relationship with reading, even if there are significant differences between the groups on the behavioural tests of reading. In other words, just because there is significant difference between DPs and CPs on a given variable, this does not mean that this variable is the underlying cause of a reading deficit in DPs. This is because a given variable may be a correlate of dyslexia which has no relationship to reading. For instance, as discussed above, Eden et al. (1996) showed, using fMRI, that DPs exhibited a visual magnocellular deficit, in contrast to CPs, but no correlation between the neuroimaging data and reading was presented in this study. Hence it is difficult to link a visual magnocellular deficit in DPs and the reading deficit in DPs reported by Eden et al. (1996). Eden et al.'s (1996) result was criticised on the grounds that the visual magnocellular deficit found in the sample of DPs in their study could be explained as a correlate, or biological marker of dyslexia, which is independent from reading (Frith and Frith, 1996). Frith and Frith (1996) also argued that such a marker could potentially be useful in the early detection of dyslexia because, according to these authors, V5/MT+ is fully myelinated before birth hence it is unlikely that its connections would change. A criticism on the grounds of 'a correlate of dyslexia' can also be put forward regarding Nicolson, Fawcett et al.'s (1999) study which revealed a significantly lower BOLD signal in adult DPs compared to CPs in the R cerebellar cortex when learning a new sequence of finger presses and when performing a pre-learned sequence of finger presses. Finally, this criticism can be made for all studies which have demonstrated structural brain differences between DPs and CPs, without any attempt at demonstrating a relationship with reading.

Showing that a given deficit (defined by the main theories of dyslexia) is found in DPs without demonstrating its relationship with a reading deficit becomes even more alarming once evidence for the presence of a given deficit in a sample with a different developmental disorder is reported. For instance, a magnocellular deficit, measured on the behavioural level was demonstrated in individuals with autism and spared reading (White et al., 2008) and children with Williams syndrome (Braddick, Atkinson, and Wattam-Bell, 2003) who develop reading skills commensurate with their verbal mental age (Laing, Hulme, Grant, and Karmiloff-Smith, 2001). Furthermore, cerebellar abnormalities were reported in ADHD (e.g., Berquin et al., 1998), schizophrenia (e.g., Nopoulos, Ceilley, Gailis, and Andreasen, 1999) and autism (e.g., Allen and Courchesne, 2003). Therefore, in the search for the underlying cause of dyslexia, studies should not only demonstrate that there is a given deficit in DPs, but also should relate the results of this deficit to DPs' reading performance.

The approach taken in the research presented in this chapter is different to the previous neuroimaging studies run within the theoretical frameworks of the main theories of dyslexia.

First, in contrast to these studies, this study does not investigate tasks designed to selectively tap into phonological, magnocellular or cerebellar functioning, but focuses on testing reading deficit - the defining deficit in this disorder. Secondly, because of the unique characteristics of the fMRI technique this chapter contrasts the predictions of the main theories of dyslexia regarding the neural correlates of reading impairment in DPs (as compared to the CPs). Thirdly, the predictions of the main theories of dyslexia, in contrast to the previous research, are tested in one sample of DPs.

Before the goals of this chapter are fully specified, however, to put them in context, a brief review of some relevant issues arising from the results on neuroimaging studies of DPs' single word and pseudoword reading is presented.

1.6. Neuroimaging Studies of Reading in Adult DPs, As Compared to CPs

Neuroimaging studies on words and pseudowords comparing DPs and CPs show functional differences between these two groups. In DPs these differences manifest as relative (in comparison with the CPs) underactivation of both the L hemisphere ventral and dorsal reading networks (e.g., Brunswick, McCrory, Price, Frith, and Frith, 1999; Paulesu et al., 2001; Pugh, Mencl, Jenner et al., 2000; Salmelin, Service, Kiesila, Uutela, and Salonen, 1996). In contrast, these also show that DPs exhibit significantly more activation than CPs in the L anterior cortex (e.g., Brunswick et al., 1999; Shaywitz et al., 1998), a finding that is usually interpreted in terms of a compensatory mechanism. More specifically, Brunswick et al. (1999) interpreted overactivation in a pre-motor region of Broca's area (BA6/44) in terms of an 'enforced use of an effortful compensatory strategy involving sublexical assembly of articulatory routines'.

Shaywitz et al. (1998) stated that the overactivation in DPs in the anterior areas 'may represent the neural consequences of the increased effort required of dyslexic readers in carrying out phonologic analysis, an increase in effort measured behaviourally as an increased error rate on tasks that make demands on such analysis'. Underactivation of the dorsal and ventral cortex is consistent with the predictions of the PDT, the overactivation for the anterior area in adult DPs is not in agreement with the PDT because as anterior areas are involved in phonological processing (please see discussion on this issue above), deficient anterior areas would be predicted by the PDT to be one of the potential sources of impaired reading in dyslexia (Hulme and Snowling, 2009). However, as pointed out earlier, a more recent meta-analysis (Maisog, Einbinder, Flowers, Turkeltaub, and Eden, 2008) revealed no support for overactivation in L frontal cortex in DPs, suggesting that these findings, are likely to be variable in spatial location and in reproducibility.

For more details on the differences between DPs' and CPs' reading of single words and pseudowords please see reviews (Demonet, Taylor, and Chaix, 2004; Frost et al., 2008; Habib, 2000; Perfetti and Bolger, 2004; Price and Mechelli, 2005; Pugh, Mencl, Jenner et al., 2000; Salmelin and Helenius, 2004; Sandak, Mencl, Frost, and Pugh, 2004; Temple, 2002).

1.6.1. Functional Connectivity Studies on Reading (Adult DPs vs CPs)

Interestingly, there have been some studies with adults on word and pseudoword reading within the framework of functional connectivity. Functional connectivity can be defined as temporal correlations between spatially remote neurophysiological events (Friston, Frith,

Liddle, and Frackowiak, 1993). It considers relationships between different brain areas that function in a cooperative manner to process information during a given cognitive task (Horwitz, Rumsey, and Donohue, 1998). For instance, Horwitz et al. (1998) reported a PET study of men with dyslexia and matched CPs. It was found that the cerebral blood flow in the L angular gyrus (BA39) in DPs showed only weak within-task and across-subject correlations (functional connectivity) with cerebral blood flow in the extrastriate occipital and temporal lobe regions during reading aloud of single words, indicating a lack of functional connectivity between these structures. In contrast, the CPs exhibited strong and significant correlations within these areas, indicative of functional connectivity. The authors concluded that dyslexia is due to a functional disconnection in the cortical reading network.

A subsequent study (Pugh, Mencl, Shaywitz et al., 2000) also investigated the functional connectivity of the angular gyrus (to BA22, medial and lateral BA18/19 and BA17). The results for a nonword rhyming task revealed that functional connectivity was disrupted in DPs between the L angular gyrus and the following areas within the L hemisphere: Wernicke's area, the lingual gyrus, the lateral extrastriate cortex and the primary visual cortex. No such disruption was observed in DPs for the single letter rhyming task (with low demand on phonological assembly). However, functional connectivity was not disrupted in the R hemisphere. The authors concluded that a phonological processing deficit underlies dyslexia and that posterior regions in the R hemisphere play a compensatory role in phonological processing in DPs. The differences in functional connectivity between DPs and CPs, on a task with high demand on phonological assembly, suggest potential differences on the behavioural measures of reading between DPs and CPs. Indeed there was a significant difference between these groups on non-word reading (the mean standard score on the Woodcock Johnson-Revised word attack test was 81 (SD=1.9) for DPs and 114 (SD=1.5) for CPs, with no overlap between the groups).

The significance of the results from the connectivity studies on adult DPs lies in the suggestion that although the ventral and dorsal systems are poorly developed in DPs, DPs' systems do not seem to be characterised by 'developmental lesions' and presumably can be altered with appropriate reading intervention (Eden et al., 2004; Shaywitz et al., 2004; see reading intervention studies by: Simos et al., 2002; Temple et al., 2003).

1.6.2. Criticisms of Neuroimaging Studies on Reading and the Approach Taken Here

Three criticisms concerning the neuroimaging studies on single word/pseudoword reading with DPs should be raised in connection with the goals of this chapter. First, the majority of the neuroimaging studies on dyslexia have been carried out within one theoretical framework, mostly the PDT, and have focused only on selected brain regions. Such an approach, although important because it allows for exploring specific brain regions, cannot provide a fuller picture of the underlying neural underpinnings of reading deficits in dyslexia. Unimpaired reading involves a network of brain areas (Price, 2000; Turkeltaub, Eden, Jones, and Zeffiro, 2002), all of which are potentially important and can impair reading when deficient. Therefore the study presented in this chapter used an ROI approach where the activation is tested in brain regions specified by the hypotheses presented below. Although such an approach has limitations (only the areas hypothesised by the three main theories of dyslexia are taken into consideration), it goes much beyond the narrower approach taken within each theoretical framework, where only the areas hypothesised by one theory were usually considered.

Second, the findings of previous studies were usually designed and interpreted within the PDT. It is interesting to mention here that such studies have also revealed significant between group differences in some other areas crucially associated with the remaining main theories, such as the cerebellum (Paulesu et al., 1996) and the primary visual cortex (Shaywitz et al., 1998). This criticism is addressed here by taking into consideration the predictions of all three main theories of dyslexia tested on the same sample of DPs.

Third, bearing in mind the large heterogeneity of DPs (Heim et al., 2008; Menghini et al., 2010; Ramus et al., 2003; Reid et al., 2007; Snowling, 2008), a comparison of individual DPs to the control group provides the opportunity to detect deficits on the neural level which otherwise could be obscured in the between group analysis due to considerable individual variability within the DP group. Despite the importance of such an approach in the dyslexia research, none of the neuroimaging studies on reading, involving fMRI, has compared individual DPs with the control group. The study reported in this chapter is the first one to take this approach.

1.7. The Aims, Stimuli and Hypotheses

The main goal of this chapter is to shed more light on the neural correlates of reading impairment in developmental dyslexia as hypothesised by the main theories of this disorder. The study presented in this chapter takes a broader ROI approach than has been used previously and places particular emphasis on a multiple case study approach to investigate individual differences among DPs, using fMRI. The comparisons involved in this study would not have been possible with PET which relies on group 'averaging'.

The predictions of the three main current theories of dyslexia are tested using words which are ecologically valid stimuli. Single words, rather than sentences or connected text, were chosen in the current study to enable comparison with previous studies (please see the section 'Neuroimaging studies of reading in DPs, as compared to CPs') and with the existing models of reading, most of which have been developed for single word/pseudoword reading. Furthermore, stimuli of this type do not introduce many complexities, such as the processing of grammar, pragmatics or the reading of text which involves eye movements and comprehension processes, all of which could potentially confound the BOLD signal, especially where comparisons between DPs and CPs are involved.

1.7.1. Hypotheses

First, if as predicted by the PDT, the neural correlates of reading deficit in DPs lie within the phonological processing network, then DPs should exhibit abnormal activation in comparison with CPs in all or some areas within this network. As can be seen from the literature review, presented above, phonological processing involves many brain areas and it is still unclear what exact role each given area plays in phonological processing. A summary of areas involved in phonological processing, together with their hypothesised functions was presented earlier. Broadly speaking, the phonological processing network includes the following areas: the L inferior frontal gyrus (BA44/45) - Broca's area, L BA22 (Wernicke's area), the L middle temporal gyrus (BA21), the L insula, L inferior parietal lobule (including the L angular gyrus (BA39) and the L supramarginal gyrus (BA40)), the L precentral gyrus PMC (Premotor cortex) (BA6) (also known as SMA), the L fusiform gyrus (BA19/37) and the L posterior fusiform gyrus. The role of the L posterior fusiform gyrus is controversial, as discussed above, with some researchers claiming that it is involved exclusively in orthographic processing (Cohen et al., 2000; Cohen et al., 2002; Cohen et al., 2003) and others (McCrory et al., 2005; Price and Devlin, 2003) that it is involved in mapping orthography on to phonology. These areas are used to test the PDT.

The phonological areas listed above are for individuals who have the L hemisphere as the language dominant one. The participants recruited for this study were screened for L-handedness (please see Method section below), as it has been demonstrated that in the vast majority of R handed persons language is L lateralised (Knecht et al., 2000).

To detect abnormality in the neural correlates of reading impairment of a given DP (as compared to the control group) not all the areas involved in phonological processing need to exhibit abnormal activation, because there may be differences between individuals in the neural implementation of the phonological network. The PDT further predicts that DPs should not show abnormal activations in magnocellular system areas - such as the V5/MT and the cerebellum, as predicted by the visual MDT and CDT, respectively.

Second, if, as predicted by the visual MDT, reading impairment in dyslexia is due to magnocellular dysfunction, then DPs should exhibit significantly lower activation (during single word reading) in comparison to CPs in the V5/MT, because this area is thought to be receiving the input predominantly from the magnocellular stream (Tootell and Taylor, 1995; Watson et al., 1993). As described above, this prediction is supported by the finding that a virtual lesion of V5/MT, created by rTMS during reading, resulted in visual errors, but not in difficulties with phonological processing. Furthermore, there should also be differences between DPs and CPs in other areas with magnocellular input, as reviewed above. In this chapter, three areas in both hemispheres are targeted: the L and R V5/MT, L and R V1, and L and R V2. This is because of reported correlations between these areas and reading performance (Demb et al., 1998), and because they can be more reliably localised than the remaining motion sensitive areas, using currently available cytoarchitectonic maps (Amunts, Malikovic, Mohlberg, Schormann, and Zilles, 2000; Malikovic et al., 2007). Underactivation in L and R V1 and/or in V2 was interpreted in support of the MDT only if found jointly with underactivation in the V5/MT. The V5/MT receives input predominantly from the magnocellular stream, but V1 and V2 consist of partially separated magno and parvo cell inputs. Hence, the underactivation of V1 and V2 may reflect underactivation of either magno cells or parvo cells, or a combination of these. A hypothetical Visual Deficit Theory (VDT) has been postulated, and it is argued that in cases which exhibit underactivation in V1 and/or V2 without hypoactivation of V5/MT, underactivation in DPs is in agreement with the VDT, but not with the visual MDT.

The V5/MT, V1 and V2 in both hemispheres were important for testing the visual MDT. This is because visual processing from the binocular zone is processed by homologous areas in both L and R hemispheres (Wurtz and Kandel, 2000) and neuroimaging studies which have investigated activation in the magnocellular system have usually tested both L and R hemisphere areas (Demb et al., 1998; Eden et al., 1996).

Third, as described above, the CDT makes clear predictions regarding the involvement of the cerebellum in reading acquisition. According to this theory the impaired cerebellum in DPs who are learning to read will lead to difficulties with reading acquisition (Nicolson et al.,

2001). However, the theory is less explicit regarding the involvement of the cerebellum in reading in adults. According to Roderick Nicolson (email communication, 1st of March 2013) the CDT would predict less cerebellar involvement in unimpaired adult reading (than in reading acquisition in a child), nevertheless it would predict some involvement of this brain structure in adult reading. This prediction is supported by the results from the neuroimaging studies in skilled adult readers, including the results from a meta-analysis of neuroimaging studies (Fulbright et al., 1999; Milne, Syngeniotis, Jackson, and Corballis, 2002; Turkeltaub et al., 2002) and a study which investigated cerebellar activation (other than sensori-motor activation related to finger movements) during Braille reading in blind participants (Gizewski, Timmann, and Forsting, 2004). Given that according to the CDT, the underlying cause of dyslexia is a cerebellar impairment, one would predict, on the basis of this theory, that it is very likely that the neural correlates of reading problems in DPs are within the cerebellum and therefore DPs, in comparison to CPs, should show abnormal activation during reading in some regions in this brain structure. However, the CDT does not specify which cerebellar areas should be affected. As the cerebellum consists of approximately 50% of all the brain neurons (Brodal, 1981) and is a heterogeneous structure, additional predictions must be made about which areas should exhibit significantly lower activation in DPs, as compared to CPs, during silent reading. As the research reported in this chapter uses a task which involves language processing, the focus here is mainly on the cerebellar language areas.

Probably the most robust results regarding the language areas in the cerebellum come from the meta-analysis by Stoodley and Schmahmann (2009), reported above. These areas include: the R Lobule VI (Hem), R and L Crus I (Hem), R Crus II (Hem), R Vermal Lobule VIIAt (R Vermal Lobule VI) and L Lobule VI (Hem). These areas were selected to test the CDT in DPs' reading. As Stoodley and Schmahmann's (2009) findings overlap with some other important cerebellar findings reported above, selecting them as ROIs would allow relation of the findings from this chapter to these earlier important findings. First, the R Vermal lobule VI was also reported by Pernet et al. (2009) as a structure which (together with the R lentiform nucleus) differentiated between DPs and CPs. Second, the R and L H Crus I, R and L H Crus II, R and L H lobule VI, and R and L H lobule VIIB significantly differed between CPs and DPs in silent reading in a study by Fulbright et al. (1999). Finally, four cerebellar areas of interest here are: the R and L H Crus II and the paramedian R and L H lobule (VIIB). This is because, as described in the Introduction, Finch et al. (2002), in a histological study of the cerebellum, found the biggest difference between the DPs and CPs (with DPs exhibiting more large Purkinje cells and fewer small Purkinje cells), in the Crus II and paramedian lobule (VIIB). This difference may indicate an abnormal representation of the head and neck, together with an abnormal representation of the articulators in DPs (Finch et al., 2002). This in turn could cause early speech problems and presumably could affect inner speech which is important for silent reading (Rayner and Pollatsek, 1989). The L H Crus II and R and L H lobule (VIIB) were not reported in Stoodley and Schmahmann's (2009) findings, however they were included as ROI because, as discussed above, cerebellar activation was noted in these lobules (among others) during unimpaired adult reading (Fulbright et al., 1999) and the biggest difference between the DPs and CPs was found in these lobules (Finch et al., 2002).

The areas chosen here as ROIs in the cerebellum are most likely best suited to assess involvement of the cerebellum in reading, as presented in the main route of the hypothetical causal ontogenetic chain (Nicolson et al., 2001). Although the experiment presented in this chapter was not set-up to investigate the involvement of the cerebellum in automatic skills, it is possible that some aspect of automaticity in reading/language processing (as specified in the non-main route of the hypothetical ontogenetic causal chain) (Nicolson et al., 2001) can also be assessed by testing the activation in the R Lobule VI (Vermis), which is included in the ROI. This is because it was suggested (Pernet et al., 2009) that this area, in connection with other areas outside the cerebellum, such as the R lentiform nucleus, is engaged in the process of automatisation of skills.

Before proceeding further, it needs to be emphasised that each theory makes unique predictions about the brain areas which underline reading impairment in DPs. Additionally, the MDT postulates that the magnocellular system is important in the acquisition of 'accurate visual representations of the written, orthographic, form of words' and that this is essential in order to grasp their structure at the phonemic level. Therefore, it has been hypothesised (Stein, 2003) that a deficient magnocellular system could be the underlying cause of deficient phonological representations and therefore of a phonological deficit. Hence it is possible that the underactivation in phonological areas (coupled with the underactivation in the V5/MT) in DPs during reading in this study is also consistent with the MDT. However, the methods used in this study do not allow for teasing apart whether the underactivation in phonological areas (co-occuring with underactivation in magnocellular areas) is 'purely phonological' or has been influenced by magnocellular malfunctioning. The underactivation in DPs in phonological areas in the presence (but not in the absence) of the underactivation of magnocellular areas is interpreted here as being consistent with the MDT (and with the PDT, as specified above). Furthermore, the CDT (Nicolson, et al., 2001) predicts that a phonological deficit (in phonological awareness and in reading) can be caused by a cerebellar impairment. Therefore it is possible that the underactivation in phonological areas (coupled with the underactivation in cerebellar areas) in DPs during reading, in the study presented here, may also be consistent with the CDT. But, the methodology used does not allow for teasing apart whether the underactivation in phonological areas is 'purely phonological' or has been influenced by cerebellar malfunctioning. The underactivation in DPs in phonological areas in the presence (but not in the absence) of the underactivation of cerebellar areas is interpreted here as being consistent with the CDT (and with the PDT, as specified above).

It is important to keep in mind that interpreting underactivation within the phonological areas as being also consistent with the CDT and the MDT, holds only if one takes the view of the CDT or the MDT, respectively. In contrast, from the theoretical perspective of the PDT such interpretations do not hold. This is because according to the PDT, the underlying cause of reading deficit in dyslexia on the biological level is within the L Perisylvian region or L temporo-parietal and L frontal region (Frith, 1997; Hulme and Snowling, 2009) and not within the magnocellular and/or cerebellar areas.

2. Method

2.1. Participants

Thirty eight students from three UK universities participated in the study. The participants were recruited via adverts posted on the student information boards in three universities. Additionally, in the case of one university the study was also advertised via website. They were all right handed, with native English, with normal, or corrected to normal, vision, normal hearing, without clinical ADHD (defined as a score<70 on ADHD D index on Conners' scales), without clinical DCD, as defined in DSM-IV, or any other known neurological or psychiatric disorder. There were indications that DP8 and DP15 may be 'at risk' of clinical DCD.

Although deviance analysis (please see Results section) revealed that DP8's and DP15's z-scores were not the highest among DPs, they were the only DPs who responded 'yes' to the question on whether their DCD difficulties significantly interfered with their everyday life. This possibly indicates that the severity of their sympthoms was higher than the severity of sympthoms in other DPs in the sample reported here. These participants were included in the study, but: 1) DCD Total measure was used as a covariate in the fMRI analysis (please see the 'Data analysis' section below and 2) the fMRI data for DP8 and DP15 were also analysed searching for possible DCD effects, please see the Results section).None of the participants reported current use of any psychoactive medication.

Three control participants (CPs) were excluded from the analysis (please see the section 'fMRI data quality control' below for more details). One DP was excluded from the study because she did not provide her dyslexia diagnosis. Eighteen individual DPs and sixteen CPs (treated as a control group) were entered into a multiple case analysis. All DPs (twelve females and six males; Mean age 21.28 years (SD=3.3)) reported a history of persistent litereacy difficulties (especially with reading), and had a formal diagnosis of developmental dyslexia by an educational psychologist (obtained within three years of taking part in this study). Twelve DPs (66.7%) reported literacy difficulties occurring in one or more first-degree relatives. The remaining six DPs were not aware of a family history of literacy difficulties. CPs (eleven females and five males; Mean age 21.38 years (SD=6.03)) had no reading and spelling difficulties or any other known psychiatric or developmental disorders.

Although DPs (treated as a group) and CPs (treated as a group) were matched on the following variables: years of education (all participants were studying at a UK university), age [U=181, p=.211], handedness, [U=116, p=.347], Verbal IQ (VIQ) [U=105.5, p=.187], Performance IQ (PIQ) [t(27.35)=-.921] and Full Scale IQ (FSIQ) [t(32)=-1.76], this was not always the case in the multiple case analysis. Therefore, age, handedness and FSIQ were used as covariates in the multiple case fMRI analysis which compared every individual DP to the control group.

2.2. Materials

A broad battery of behavioural measures is needed to capture a range of effects associated with dyslexia. Tests used here can be classified in the following categories: general psychometrics, literacy measures, phonological processing (awareness and fluency) and orthographic processing. Because it is possible that the reading and spelling skills of DPs become compensated in adulthood, a set of widely used literacy measures was employed to investigate how the performance of each individual DP on literacy tests compared to CPs' performance around the time of the fMRI reading study.

2.2.1. General Psychometrics, ADHD and DCD

2.2.1.1. The Edinburgh Handedness Inventory

This instrument (Oldfield, 1971) consists of a list of 10 questions which investigate direction and strength of hand preference in 10 everyday activities. The dependent variable was handedness index, calculated according to the following equation:

$$H = \frac{(R-L)}{(R+L)} * 100\%$$

where H denotes handedness, R is the number of checks assigned by a participant to the actions performed with the right hand and L is the number checks assigned by a participant to the actions performed with the left hand.

2.2.1.2. Intelligence Tests

All DPs in the study had recent dyslexia assessment reports. To avoid practice effects due to repetition of IQ testing, an IQ test was not administered to DPs and the scores were taken from their psychological assessment reports. This is considered as common practice because IQ measures are relatively stable across lifespan, with scores collected in earlier life used to predict educational outcome and employment prospects in later years (McCall, 1977). All IQ scores for DPs were from the Wechsler Adult Intelligence Scale - III (WAIS-III) (Wechsler, 1997).

IQ scores for CPs were obtained using the Wechsler Abbreviated Scale of Intelligence (WASI) (Wechsler, 1999), which consists of two verbal subtests (vocabulary and similarities) and two performance subtests (block design and matrix reasoning). Variables here were: FSIQ, VIQ and PIQ. No participants with the FSIQ lower than the average score (90) were included in the study.

2.2.1.3. ADHD Measure

As discussed in the Introduction, ADHD shows higher rates of comorbidity with dyslexia than expected by chance (Gilger, Pennington, and DeFries, 1992) and it was found to mediate various deficits in developmental dyslexia, such as between-group differences in postural sway and reading (Fergusson and Horwood, 1992; Reid and Hansen, 2013; Rochelle, Witton, and Talcott, 2009). Therefore, Conners' Adult ADHD Rating Scale (CAARS-Self-Report, Screening Version: 30 questions) (Conners, Erhardt, and Sparrow, 1999) was used to screen the participants.

Four indexes were obtained: ADHD Index (D) (designed to identify the adults in a population who are likely to be diagnosed with clinical ADHD), Inattention (A), Hyperactivity/Impulsivity (B) and Combined ADHD Score (A+B) (an index which combines both scores of Inattention (A) and Hyperactivity/Impulsivity (B)). The exclusion criterion was a T-score above 70 on the ADHD Index (D). The reason for this cut-off point is that a T-score above 70 indicates that an individual is likely to have significant levels of symptoms that may meet the DSM-IV diagnostic criteria for clinical ADHD (Conners et al., 1999).

2.2.1.4. DCD (Also Known As Developmental Dyspraxia)

The questionnaire used was based on the DSM-IV (APA, 1994), the questions in the Adult DCD Checklist provided by the Dyspraxia Foundation and Developmental Adult Neuro-Diversity Association (DANDA) and questions devised by A. A. Reid (which provide more detailed information on gross and fine motor coordination). It consisted of five parts: 1) motor-coordination problems throughout early development (five questions), 2) gross motor coordination difficulties (nine questions), 3) fine motor coordination difficulties (sixteen questions), 4) the DSM-IV (APA, 1994) questions on whether motor coordination deficit significantly interferes with academic achievement or activities of daily living (four questions) and 5) the DSM-IV (APA, 1994) question on any other medical conditions which could cause or increase motor coordination difficulties. Including this questionnaire into the test battery had two aims. First, as DCD was found to co-occur with dyslexia (Portwood, 2000), any participant who was likely to have significant levels of symptoms that meet the DSM-IV (APA, 1994) diagnostic criteria for clinical DCD, was excluded from the study reported here. (DP8 and DP15 may have been 'at risk' of DCD, please see the sections Participants and Results). Second, as adult DPs sometimes report difficulties with gross and fine motor coordination, more detailed questions about these problems were administered to collect richer profiles of the participants. One point was given for every question answered positively, denoting the presence of a difficulty. Dependent variables were: the total number of motor coordination problems throughout early development (max.=5), the number of gross motor coordination difficulties (max.=9), the number of fine motor coordination difficulties (max.=16) and a total score on motor coordination disorder (collapsing across the three categories detailed above) (max.=30).

2.2.1.5. Revised Adult Dyslexia Check List (ADCL)

A shortened version of the revised version of the ADCL was administered. It was derived from the 20-item version (Vinegrad, 1994) and consists of 12 questions which are the best at predicting dyslexia (Vinegrad, 1994). The dependent variable was the number of positive responses which indicated difficulties.

2.2.2. Literacy Tests

2.2.2.1. Single Word Reading TOWRE (Torgesen, Wagner, and Rashotte, 1999)

TOWRE (The Test of Word Reading Efficiency) (Torgesen et al., 1999), which measures reading fluency (by assessing speed) and accuracy using relatively high frequency single words, was administered. As this test only has norms up to 24.11 years and the age range of the participants in the study reported here was from 18 to 42 years, normalised scores were not used. The dependent variable was based on the raw score for the number of words read aloud correctly from the Sight Word Efficiency Form A in 45 seconds. List 'A' presented one hundred and four words. Each correctly read word was given a score of '1', hence the maximum raw score was 104.

2.2.2.2. Single Pseudoword Reading (TOWRE) (Torgesen Et Al., 1999)

The dependent variable was based on the raw score (for the same reason as for single word reading) for the number of pseudowords read aloud correctly from the Phonemic Decoding Efficiency Form A in 45 seconds. The accuracy of pronunciation was judged according to the key provided in the test. Participants' performance was also recorded and the pronunciation was double-checked by an English native speaker.

2.2.2.3. English Pseudowords (Castles and Coltheart, 1993)

The test consisted of 30 English pseudowords. The dependent variables were: percent correct and time taken to read all the items.

2.2.2.4. English Irregular Words (Castles and Coltheart, 1993)

The test consisted of 30 English irregular words. The dependent variables were: percent correct and time taken to read all the items.

2.2.2.5. WRAT3 Spelling (Wilkinson, 1993) (Blue Sheet)

One point was given for each correctly spelled word; the maximum score was 40. The dependent variable was percent correct.

2.2.3. Phonological Awareness Tests

2.2.3.1. Spoonerism Test (Brunswick et al., 1999)

As no standardised Spoonerism test for adults in English was known, the test reported by Brunswick et al. (1999) was used. It consisted of 12 word pairs, e.g. *basket, lemon*. The dependent variables were percent correct and time needed to create Spoonerisms between all the word pairs (e.g. *lasket, bemon*). The maximum raw score was 12.

2.2.3.2. Phonological Pseudoword Forced-Choice Test (Olson, Forsberg, Wise, and Rack, 1994)

This is a computerised test of phonological skill adapted from Olson, et al. (1994), which is based on silent phonological decoding. The test contained 64 trials (including four practice ones). Each trial consisted of a triplet of pseudowords, e.g. *pake, kake, dake* and participants needed to determine (by pressing one of the three response keys), which of the items sounded like a real English word (in the example given above *kake* sounds like the real English word *cake*). This task minimised the input of orthographic processing to the determination of the correct answer since all the items needed to be decoded and compared with the phonological representation of the items in the lexicon. The dependent variables were: percent correct and mean RT in milliseconds (calculated for all trials, except for the practice trials). Participants were encouraged to respond as fast as possible, while being as accurate as possible.

2.2.3.3. Phonological Fluency Tests

Random Automatised Naming (RAN) tests for colours, pictures, digits and letters (Forms A and B) from the Comprehensive Test of Phonological Processing (CTOPP) (Wagner, Torgesen, and Rashotte, 1999) were used. The dependent variable was the sum of the time (in seconds) necessary to name all the items in a given category on forms A and B. Both forms (A and B) were administered (using standard administration and scoring) because according to the manual each RAN test consists of 72-items (36 items per form) (Wagner et al., 1999).

2.2.3.4. Orthographic Processing

The Orthographic Word-Pseudohomophone Choice test (Olson et al., 1994) was used. The test contained 88 trials (including eight practice ones). Each trial consisted of a pseudohomophone pair, e.g. *rain* and *rane*. Participants had to indicate, by pressing an appropriate response key, which item was a real English word (i.e., *rain*). The rationale behind this task is that, although there may occur some automatic phonological processing (which would yield the same output for both items), the task biases towards orthographic processing because in order to make a decision, the participant has to base it on their memory of the target word's specific orthographic form. The dependent variables were percent correct and mean RT in milliseconds (calculated for all trials, except for the practice trials).

2.2.4. Stimuli and fMRI Task

There were three conditions in the fMRI experiment reported here. Condition 1 consisted of 100 real English words (high familiarity, high imageability, high concreteness, two-syllable, five to seven letters, with regular spelling as far as possible, selected using the rules on the structure of English orthography (Venezky, 1970) from the MRC Psycholinguistic Database (Coltheart, 1981)). Condition 2 contained 100 pseudowords created by the substitution of consonants in the onset or middle of real English words (used in Condition 1). They were all pronounceable pseudowords - in line with English orthography and phonology. Condition 3 (the control condition) consisted of 100 fixation crosses.

The fMRI experiment had an event-related design with stimuli from all conditions randomly intermixed, to avoid potential strategic effects. Each stimulus was displayed for 1000 milliseconds, with an SOA of 4000 milliseconds and an ISI 3000 milliseconds.

The words and pseudowords were pre-tested in a behavioural pilot experiment with five DPs and four CPs (the groups did not take part in the fMRI experiment). The task was the same as in the fMRI study, except it involved reading aloud, so that reading errors could be recorded. The items which produced errors were excluded from the stimulus set. Furthermore, the stimulus display time which ensured comfortable reading presentation time for both groups was derived from this pilot experiment. A comfortable reading speed in both groups is crucial for this task because then the potential differences in fMRI activation between an individual DP and CPs are less likely to be due to quantitative than qualitative differences in reading. It should be noted here that this chapter focuses on real word reading which involves the contrast of Conditions 1 and 3.

2.2.5. fMRI Data Acquisition

The fMRI data were acquired at the Aston University MRI Research Centre (located in Aston Day Hospital) using a 3T Trio Siemens Scanner equipped with echo planar imaging and a standard 8 channel head coil. Forty four (3 x 3 x 3 mm) slices, covering the whole brain, were acquired every 3 sec (*TR=3000 ms, TE=30, flip angle=90, FOVread=192, FOVphase=100*) for a total of 404 volumes. Within the scanning environment, the participants viewed the stimuli presented in the middle of the screen (one item per trial) in black letters on a white background. Presentation was through a mirror mounted on the head coil, placed for viewing a projection screen at the back of the MRI scanner. The participants were asked to keep their gaze fixed on the '+' sign shown on the screen (this appeared at a fixed position in the centre of the field of view). They were asked to silently read words, ensuring that they did not make any movement with their lips or mouth.

To ensure that participants did their best, they were asked to read every item as carefully as possible, because there would be a post-test after the experiment. It was explained to the participants that they should not try to memorise the words because careful reading would be sufficient for the test.

The reason the silent reading task was chosen was twofold. First, there is evidence that the cerebellum is involved in reading aloud (Price, 2000; Turkeltaub et al., 2002), which to at least a certain extent, could be accounted for by articulatory movements when pronouncing words. Here the aim was to only test other potential involvement of the cerebellum in reading. Second, it was desirable to avoid participants processing their own voice because it causes activation within the temporal areas (Price, Moore, and Frackowiak, 1996).

To monitor participants' vigilance in the scanner, they were required to press a response button (with their left index finger) when a black star (displayed during ISI) became red. This change occurred on 30 trials (10%). The participants were also asked to stay as still as possible throughout the whole fMRI session.

2.2.6. fMRI Data Pre-Processing and Analysis

2.2.6.1. Data Preprocessing

SPM5 (Statistical Parametric Mapping) software was used to preprocess (and analyse) the fMRI data. The pre-processing involved: slice timing correction, realignment, coregistration, segmentation, normalisation and smoothing (Friston, 2002).

Realignment, rather than slice timing correction, is usually the first step in the pre-processing of the data, however, because at the Aston MRI Research Centre each volume is acquired in slices in an interleaved fashion, starting from the bottom slice, it was advisable to run the slice timing correction in the first step, instead of realignment (John Ashburner, email communication, 4th of June, 2007).

A serious confound, especially in fMRI studies, can arise from changes in signal intensity over time due to head motion. The 'realign' function in SPM5 was used to remove these confounds from the fMRI data. In this study the middle slice was chosen as the reference image for realignment. Realignment parameters were saved for each participant for each session and incorporated into the design matrix as covariates (please see the 'fMRI data quality control' and Results sections below).

A coregistration function was used to coregister the functional and the structural data so as to maximise their mutual information. A segmentation function was used to segment the structural image according to tissue probability, using default maps, creating white and grey matter images and a bias-field corrected structural image.

The data were pooled into the same anatomical space as if the acquired data had been caused by a canonical brain (identical for all participants) using a spatial normalisation function. Because participants' brains vary, a spatial normalisation was then necessary to make the canonical brain assumption hold. The spatial normalisation function in SPM5, spatially normalises MRI images into a standard space defined by template images. There are two main uses for normalisation: 1) precise characterisation of functional anatomy and 2) averaging between participants (Ashburner and Friston, 1997).SPM5 provides the template images which correspond to the space defined by the International Consortium for Brain Mapping (ICBM), NIH P-20 project. They approximate the space as described in Talairach and Tournoux's co-planar stereotaxic atlas (Talairach and Tournoux, 1988).

To limit the noise and effects caused by residual differences in gyral and functional anatomy when averaging across participants, a smoothing function was used. It involves smoothing image volumes with a Gaussian kernel of a given width. More specifically, there are three reasons why data should be smoothed (Friston, 2002). First, it makes the distribution of errors more normal and ensures a good basis for the validity of the inferential statistics. Second, within the SPM5 framework, the inferences about regional effects are based on Gaussian random field theory which is based on a premise that the error terms are a plausible representation of a smooth Gaussian field. Therefore, voxels which are usually relatively large need to be smoothed. Third, the data need to be smoothed when analysis requires inter-subject averaging, as is the case of the control group, presented in this chapter. The data were smoothed with an 8 mm Gaussian kernel.

2.2.6.2. fMRI Data Quality Control

Following the recommendations by Poldrack et al. (2008), a data quality control procedure was employed. Head motion was assessed individually for each participant by examining the output from the Realignment procedure in SPM5 in the preprocessing stage. The fMRI data for three participants who had unusually large head movement (>5 mm for Translation and/or 5 degrees for Rotation), and which could not be salvaged using the recommended techniques (Poldrack, Mumford, and Nichols, 2011), were excluded from the analysis. Despite spatial realignment, residual movement-related artefacts in the fMRI data can usually be found concentrated near the edge of the brain (The FIL Methods Group, 2006). Therefore, the realignment parameters from this study were entered into the design matrix as multiple regressors, so that the residual participant's movement could be co-varied out, reducing the residual error, and improving the statistics for the investigated effects. As a further precaution fMRI data were also visually inspected for artefacts due to high signal loss. No participants were excluded on this criterion.

2.2.6.3. Data Analysis

Two types of analysis were run. A first level (fixed effect) analysis and a second level-(random effect) analysis. In the first level analysis (which implements a within-subject analysis), the Word Condition was explicitly modelled. The Fixation Cross (Control Condition) was implicitly modelled (Glaser, 2006). To avoid confounding the BOLD response due to the 'Star' stimulus (which appeared during the ISI) and 'Button Press' they were included in the design matrix as regressors.

The shape of the canonical Haemodynamic Response Function (HRF) is in line with the haemodynamic response that is normally observed and this is the default in SPM5. Further inclusion of the time and dispersion derivatives was necessary to account for variations in voxel-to-voxel and subject-to-subject responses, especially in the experiment that involved DPs, characterised by heterogeneity with respect to behavioural and neuroimaging findings.

The time derivative allows for the variation in the peak response of plus or minus one second, whereas the dispersion derivative allows for the variation in the width of the response by a similar amount (Friston, 2002).

As noted earlier, this chapter focuses on word reading which involves the contrast of Condition 1 and Condition 3. A t-contrast (Word>Fixation Cross) was probed in the first level analysis. The second level analysis involved comparison of a given individual DP and the CPs (treated as a group). In the second level analysis the error variance is calculated using the subject-to-subject variability of estimates from the first level and it enables generalisations to be made from these findings to the population from which the subjects were sampled (Friston, 2002). Data analysis in the second level involved a two-sample t-test. Two contrasts were tested: CPs>DP (to probe the underactivation in a given DP) and DP>CPs (to test the overactivation in a given DP).

Although, as described earlier, DPs were screened for cases with clinical ADHD and DCD, a number of DPs exhibited elevated scores on the ADHD and DCD measures, when compared to the CPs. Therefore ADHD A+B and DCD Total were entered into the second level analysis as covariates. Participants' performance on the post-test (please see the section 'fMRI Data Acquisition' above) was summarised in a discriminability index - *d Prime* which was calculated according to the following formula:

d Prime = Z FA – Z Hit,

where *Z FA* stands for a Z score for false alarms (signal absent, response 'yes') and a *Z Hit* stands for a Z score for hits (signal present and response 'yes'). *d Prime* (together with age, handedness and FSIQ, as discussed in the Participants section) were entered into the 2nd level analysis as covariates.

2.2.6.4. ROI Analysis (Mask)

There is now growing evidence that different brain areas, such as BA44, BA45 are characterised by high inter-participant structural variability (Amunts et al., 2004). This variability manifests in differences in the sulcal pattern, shape and size of areas, and in the relationship of area borders to surrounding sulci (Amunts et al., 2004).

Bearing in mind this inter-participant variability of brain areas, a mask for the ROI analysis was prepared using mainly cytoarchitectonic areas from the AT V. 1.8 (Eickhoff et al., 2005). The AT enables the comparison of cytoarchitecture and function, providing a routine, standardised application of probabilistic cytoarchitectonic maps as an anatomical reference for functional activations (Eickhoff et al., 2005). In contrast to classical cytoarchitectonic maps e.g., Brodmann's maps, probabilistic cytoarchitectonic maps provide stereotaxic information on the variability of cortical areas and the location in the MNI reference space (Amunts and Zilles, 2001; Zilles et al., 2002). Probabilistic cytoarchitectonic maps are based on the observer independent analysis of the cytoarchitecture in a sample of 10 human post-mortem brains, so 50% denotes that a given voxel was assigned to a given cytoarchitectonic area in 5 out of 10 brains. However, some subsequent studies used more than 10 human post-mortem brains which influences probability calculations.

Probabilistic cytoarchitectonic maps have been published for various, but not all, brain regions. Because of the hypotheses put forward in the current study (please see Introduction), the following cytoarchitectonic maps were used to create the mask: *L Area 44/L Area 45* (Amunts et al., 1999) (equivalent to Broca's area L BA44 and L BA45), *L Areas Ig1, Ig2, Id1* - the posterior insula (Kurth et al., 2009), *L Area 6* (the pre-motor cortex, equivalent to L BA6) (Geyer, 2003), *L IPC PFop, L IPC L PFt, L IPC PF, L IPC PFm,* and *L IPC PFcm* (inferior parietal lobule, these areas approximately cover the region of L BA40 on the supramarginal gyrus with extension into the depth of the Sylvian fissure (Caspers et al., 2008)); *L IPC PGa* and *IPC PGp* (Caspers et al., 2006) (inferior parietal cortex - these areas are located approximately at the position of the angular gyrus (BA39)), *L Area TE3* in the lateral part of the superior temporal gyrus, perhaps homologous to BA22 (Wernicke's area) (Morosan, Schleicher, Amunts, and Zilles, 2005), the *L hOC5* and *R hOC5* (Malikovic et al., 2007) (equivalent to L and R V5/MT), *L* and *R Area 17* and *Area 18* (Amunts et al., 2000) (equivalent to L and R V1 and V2) and nine cerebellar regions (*L Lobule VIIa Crus I (Hem), R Lobule VIIa Crus I (Hem), L Lobule VIIa Crus II (Hem), R Lobule VIIa Crus II (Hem), L Lobule VI (Hem), R Lobule VI (Hem), R Lobule VI (Vermis), L Lobule VIIb (Hem)* and *R Lobule VIIb (Hem)* (Diedrichsen, Balsters, Flavell, Cussans, and Ramnani, 2009)).

As no maps are available in the AT (V.1.8) for the entire *middle temporal gyrus* and *fusiform gyrus*, these were prepared in MarsBar (version 0.43) (Brett, Anton, Valabregue, and Poline, 2002) which relies on macroanatomically defined brain regions (Tzourio-Mazoyer et al., 2002) and therefore the results involving these areas may be less reliable. The ROI mask consisted of 31 areas. Twenty nine areas were created as individual ROIs in the AT (V.1.8) and two areas were created as individual ROIs in MarsBar (version 0.43). The ROIs created in MarsBar were coregistered (with the reslice option in SPM5) to the ROIs created in the AT (V.1.8). All ROIs were combined (and binarised) into one mask using SPM5. The thirty-one ROI mask was coregistered in SPM5 (using the reslice option) to the functional data before running the ROI analysis.

The activations found in this study, within the regions defined by the mask, were labelled using the 'Local maxima labelling' option in the AT (V.1.8). The anatomical location of a given maximum can be determined using the AT (V.1.8) by finding out: 1) whether it is assigned to a cytoarchitectonic area in the maximum probability map (MPM) and 2) what the probabilities of cytoarchitectonic areas at that position are (please see Appendix B, Tables 1-18). The MPM is defined as a summary map which was computed by the AT (V.1.8) from all currently available probabilistic maps. It defines the most likely cytoarchitectonic area at each voxel ('maximum probability map').

It has to be borne in mind here that the resolution of the functional images (normally 2–4 mm voxel size after re-sampling during spatial normalization) is lower than the spatial resolution of the probabilistic maps (1 mm voxel size). Hence, it is possible that the directly corresponding voxel may underestimate or overestimate the anatomical probabilities. To increase the reliability of the anatomical labelling, the probability at the corresponding voxel and the probability range for the surrounding voxels are calculated by the AT (V.1.8) (Eickhoff et al., 2005) (please see Appendix B, Tables 1-18).

As the fMRI analysis reported here involved DPs who were potentially characterised by considerable variability, activation in an area was considered as supporting a given hypothesis when the probability that a given voxel belonged to a given area was 10% or higher (Heim et al., 2010).

The cerebellar atlas (Diedrichsen et al., 2009) used in this study differed from the one used in the meta-analysis by Stoodley and Schmahmann (2009). Therefore the local maxima in the cerebellum reported by Stoodley and Schmahmann (2009), were relabelled and for the same coordinates slightly different labels were used in this study (please see Table 1 for details).

Table 1. Labels, obtained from the Anatomy Toolbox (Eickhoff et al., 2005) used in this study for coordinates provided by Stoodley and Schmahmann (2009)

MNI coordinates	Stoodley and Schmahmann's (2009) labels	Labels used in this study
36 - 62 - 28	R lobule VI	R Lobule VIIa Crus I (Hem) (probability: 66% (10-66%)) R Lobule VI (Hem) (probability: 34% (34-90%))
34 - 82 - 36	R Crus I	R Lobule VIIa Crus I (Hem) (probability: 89% (78-98%))
14 - 86 - 34	R Crus I/II	R Lobule VIIa CrusII (Hem) (probability: 60% (17-82%)) R Lobule VIIa Crus I (Hem) (probability: 38% (18-80%))
4 - 82 - 26	R lobule VIIAt	R Lobule VI (vermis) (probability: 88% (29-88%))
-42 - 58 - 26	L lobule VI	L Lobule VI (Hem) (probability: 32% (3-32%)) L Lobule VIIa Crus I (Hem) (probability: 44% (44-94%))

2.3. Procedure

The study obtained local ethics committee approval. Prior to taking part in the study, participants were informed about the procedures to be used and that the collected data were confidential and anonymous. Written informed consent to participate in the study was given by all the participants. The research presented in this chapter was carried out in accordance with the ethical standards of the British Psychological Society and approved by the Human Sciences Ethics Committee at Aston University, UK.

2.3.1. Behavioural Testing

Every participant was tested individually in a quiet room. Each session lasted approximately 2 hours. All published tests were administered according to the instructions given in the manuals. The effects of the order of tests was not controlled for, however, the order of tests was reversed for half of each group of participants. Olson's Orthographic Word-Pseudohomophone Choice test (Olson et al., 1994) and the Phonological Pseudoword Forced-Choice test (Olson et al., 1994) were run using SuperLab V.2 on a Dell Pentium 4 PC with a RB-410/RB-610 response box (Cedrus Corporation).

2.3.2. fMRI Testing

Before going into the scanner, participants read instructions and completed a practice run of exactly the same task as they were going to do in the scanning environment, but with different stimuli, to avoid repetition effects. It was ensured that every participant understood and was able to do the task before they started the fMRI session.

Participants were positioned head first and supine in the scanner. Testing in the scanner involved, first running seven dummy scans to obtain equilibrium, second - obtaining a structural high resolution MRI image, third running the reading experiment (approximately 20 minutes). The whole MR scanning session took approximately 45 minutes.

Participants completed the post-test after they left the scanner. The post-test consisted of 64 items: 32 of these items occurred in the fMRI experiment and 32 items were not presented in the fMRI experiment. Participants were asked to read every item and decide (by pressing an appropriate button) whether they saw a given item in the fMRI experiment. The items which were not present in the fMRI experiment had the same characteristics as the items presented in the experiment. The post-test was used to ensure that participants did their best at reading the stimuli. Their scores were summarised in a discriminability index - *d Prime* (please see the section 'Data analysis' above) and entered as a covariate into the 2nd level neuroimaging analysis.

Presentation of the stimuli for the practice session, the experimental run in the scanner and the post-test was via Presentation software (Version 10.3: Neurobehavioural Systems). Both the practice and the post-test were run on a Dell Celeron laptop and the task in the scanner on a Dell Pentium 4 PC.

3. Results

3.1. DPs' Individual Performance on the Psychometric Measurements

The deficits in information processing associated with dyslexia are usually characterised by considerable heterogeneity. Group analyses can therefore obscure the importance of individual deficits at the group level. A multiple case study approach was therefore adopted in this chapter. A multiple case study is a more detailed study of individual cases, compared to a control group (Ramus et al., 2003; Reid et al., 2007; White et al., 2006).

For a detailed description of the tests and measurements used, please see the Method section. Within the individual case study approach, measures for a given DP, were converted to z-scores (please see Table 2, Table 3 and Table 4 below), with reference to the mean and the SD of the control group. The equation used to calculate z-scores is shown below.

$$z = \frac{y_{\mathrm{dp}} - x_{\mathrm{cg}}}{SD_{\mathrm{cg}}}$$

where z denotes z-score; y_{dp} denotes raw score of an individual participant with dyslexia; x_{cg} denotes mean of the control group; SD_{cg} denotes standard deviation of the control group.

The z-scores for each DP and mean and SD scores for the CPs are reported in Tables 2-4. For some tests, individual z-scores were averaged across relevant measures to yield composite scores. These composite variables are independent - the measures used for a given composite variable are not used in any other composite variable.

As averaging several imperfectly correlated z-scores resulted in composites which, for the control group, had a mean of zero but reduced standard deviations (<1), the composite scores were re-standardised by dividing them by the standard deviation of the control group (Ramus et al., 2003). These re-standardised z-scores are reported as composite scores. Composite scores (marked in Italics in Table 2, Table 3 and Table 4) were calculated for the following measures: PSEUDOWORD READING and IRREGULAR WORD READING (please see Table 3); PHONOLOGICAL AWARENESS, PHONOLOGICAL FLUENCY and ORTHOGRAPHY (please see Table 4).

Abnormal performance was defined as $z \leq -1.65$, which corresponds to performance at or below the 5th percentile. The 5th percentile was used in previous multiple-case studies to define deviant performance (e.g., Ramus et al., 2003; Reid et al., 2007; White et al., 2006). Negative z-scores denote performance that is worse than that of the control group.

There was no need to calculate a composite score for word reading because only one measure was collected using the TOWRE test. TOWRE performance relies mostly on higher frequency words that are well known to the participants. PSEUDOWORD READING consisted of the following measures: number of pseudowords read correctly (TOWRE) and percent correct and reading time for the Pseudoword reading test (Castles and Coltheart, 1993). IRREGULAR WORD READING (Castles and Coltheart, 1993) consisted of irregular word reading percent correct and reading time.

PHONOLOGICAL AWARENESS consisted of the following measures: Spoonerisms time, Spoonerisms percent correct, Phonological Pseudoword Forced-Choice test (Olson et al., 1994) RT and percent correct. These measures were combined because they involve the appreciation that phonological representations of words/pseudowords consist of smaller units – phonemes. PHONOLOGICAL FLUENCY consisted of time for RAN Colour, Picture, Digit and Letter (CTOPP) (Wagner et al., 1999). Finally, ORTHOGRAPHY consisted of the Orthographic Word-Pseudohomophone Choice test (Olson et al., 1994) percent correct and RT.

Composite variables were not calculated for ADHD and DCD because some measures overlapped (e.g. ADHD D overlapped with, for instance, ADHD A+B and the DCD Total overlapped with every other measure of DCD), and therefore would violate the assumption that a composite variable is computed from independent measures of the same construct. Most ADHD measures (please see Table 2) are given as T-scores. DCD scores are raw scores because they were not based on a standardised test. Every DP was compared on ADHD A+B and all measures of DCD to CPs using the z-score calculated according to the equation given above. It was demonstrated (Willcutt and Pennington, 2000) that reading difficulties are most strongly associated with the inattentive sub-type of ADHD, but also, albeit less strongly with the hyperactive sub-type. Therefore, the ADHD A+B measure, which includes both ADHD types, was chosen as a covariate in the fMRI analysis. The results could also potentially be confounded by the fact that some DPs exhibited z-scores ≤ -1.65 on DCD measures (please see Table 2). As DCD Total score gave the best overall summary measure of DCD, it was used as the covariate in the fMRI analysis.

Focusing on the general psychometric measures, all but two DPs (DP5 and DP16) scored ≤ -1.65 on the Adult Dyslexia Check List (Vinegrad, 1994), indicating that they experienced significantly more dyslexia-related difficulties than CPs (please see Table 2). The screening procedure for this study ensured that no DP had an FSIQ score<90; therefore only DPs with average or above FSIQ scores were included in the study. Most scores on FSIQ were 'average', seven DPs (DP1, DP2, DP4, DP7, DP10, DP13 and DP16) were 'high average' and one (DP5) was 'superior'. Similarly, most scores on PIQ were 'average', one (DP16) was 'high average' and three DPs (DP5, DP7 and DP13) were 'superior'. The scores for VIQ were characterised by more variability, with DP17 exhibiting a 'borderline', DP14 the 'low average', eight DPs (DP3, DP6, DP8, DP9, DP11, DP13, DP15 and DP18) 'average', seven

DPs (DP2, DP4, DP5, DP7, DP10, DP12 and DP16) 'high average' and one (DP1) 'superior' scores. Because the core deficits in dyslexia are in the language domain (Hulme and Snowling, 2009), scores on VIQ may be significantly lower in adult DPs than in the control group (Ramus et al., 2003).

It is interesting to note that despite screening participants for being 'at risk' of clinical ADHD', six (33%) DPs (DP2, DP3, DP7, DP9, DP15 and DP18) revealed ADHD (A+B) z-scores equal to or higher than 1.65 SD below the mean of CPs (please see Table 2). This means that although they did not meet the criteria for clinical ADHD, they did exhibit more ADHD characteristics than CPs. Furthermore, 11 (66.7%) DPs (DP1, DP2, DP3, DP7, DP9, DP10, DP11, DP12, DP14, DP15 and DP18) exhibited DCD Total z-scores equal to or more than 1.65 SD below the mean of the CPs. All six participants who had composite scores 1.65 SD below the mean of controls on ADHD were also impaired on DCD. There was a relatively large overlap of symptoms, even when the diagnosis was controlled for, especially with regard to the symptoms of DCD.

The issue of the comorbidity of ADHD and DCD with dyslexia is an important one because it may be a potential confound in the analyses. Confounds could arise from the distinctive characteristics of a given disorder (e.g., an inappropriate and persistent pattern of inattention and/or hyperactivity and impulsivity (ADHD) and impairment in the development of motor coordination (DCD) (American Psychiatric Association, 1994)), as well as the overlapping characteristics (e.g., speed of processing deficits (ADHD and dyslexia (Shanahan et al., 2006; Willcutt, Pennington, Olson, Chhabildas, and Hulslander, 2005)) and the tendency to lose place while reading (DCD and dyslexia) (Dyspraxia Foundation, 2012; Reid et al., 2007)).

In the study reported in this chapter, six DPs (33.3%) exhibited ADHD (A+B) z-scores equal to or more than 1.65 SD below the mean of CPs. This is a lower occurrence than in Kaplan et al.'s (1998) study, however, it has to be borne in mind that in the study reported here, no DPs who exhibited clinical ADHD and DCD were included in this study (although there were indications that DP8 and DP15 may be 'at risk' of clinical DCD). Difficulty in recruiting dyslexics without ADHD characteristics may be due to the shared genetic risk factors that underlie both these disorders (please see Introduction).

There is growing evidence that reading-impaired individuals exhibit difficulties in motor control (Denckla, 1985; Fawcett and Nicholson, 1995; Haslum, 1989; Iversen et al., 2005; McPhillips and Sheehy, 2004; Miles, 1993; Wolff et al., 1984). Kaplan et al. (1998) reported that 63% of their reading-disabled children also met the criteria for DCD. In the current study, however, two DPs (11.1%) were identified as possibly being 'at risk' of DCD. In contrast, ten DPs (55.6%) exhibited DCD-type difficulties of a 'sub-clinical' nature.

With respect to performance of DPs on real word, irregular word, and pseudoword reading and spelling, as revealed by the composite and z-scores summarised in Table 3, 11 DPs (DP2, DP3, DP4, DP8, DP9, DP12, DP13, DP14, DP15, DP16 and DP17), (61%) exhibited a deficit across all the measures; two cases (DP7 and DP10) (11%) showed a deficit on real word reading, pseudoword reading, and spelling; one case (DP11) (5.6%) on pseudoword reading and spelling; one case (DP18) (5.6%) on irregular word and pseudoword reading and spelling; one case (DP6) (5.6%) just on spelling; finally two cases (DP1 and DP5) (11%) show no deficits on these variables.

All, but two DPs (88.9%) were impaired on spelling and all DPs, except three DPs (83.3%) on the pseudoword reading composite. Furthermore, DPs exhibited the largest impairments on these two measures.

Table 2. Individual performance of DPs on the general psychometric tests

Measures/ Participant number	1	2	3	4	5	6	7	8	9	10	11	12	13	14	15	16	17	18	Controls
Age	27	20	21	19	31	22	18	25	19	20	23	20	19	20	19	20	20	20	21.4 (6.0)
Handedness	30	55.6	90	100	70	100	100	64.7	70	90	83.3	80	86.7	86	100	100	70	78	84.8 (21.4)
VIQ SS	121	119	97	114	116	108	112	107	106	117	96	111	97	88	101	114	79	108	111.5 (6.6)
PIQ SS	107	102	105	109	124	102	120	106	94	104	105	106	127	98	90	110	108	107	110.4 (12.7)
FSIQ SS	116	112	100	114	121	106	118	107	101	112	100	109	110	91	97	114	92	108	112.4 (9.0)
ADHDD@	57	63	58	53	59	55	57	57	57	57	58	58	48	53	55	34	48	63	50.6 (5.3)
ADHDA@	74	78	77	56	56	64	85	56	79	63	60	65	56	54	66	51	45	72	56.8 (9.8)
ADHDB@	70	61	66	55	64	54	51	50	59	48	55	48	45	57	59	39	57	68	49.6 (7.3)
ADHD (A+B)@	64	73	77	57	62	61	72	54	74	57	59	58	51	57	66	44	51	73	54.4 (6.8)
ADHD (A+B)*	-1.4	**-2.7**	**-3.3**	-0.4	-1.1	-1.0	**-2.6**	0.1	**-2.9**	-0.4	-0.7	-0.5	0.5	-0.4	**-1.7**	1.5	0.5	**-2.7**	n/a
ADCL*	**-4.7**	**-6.2**	**-3.9**	**-5.5**	-0.1	**-2.4**	**-3.9**	**-2.4**	**-7.8**	**-7.0**	**-3.2**	**-4.7**	**-2.4**	**-5.5**	**-4.7**	-1.6	**-4.7**	**-3.2**	0.9 (1.3)
DCD (Early dev.)*	**-3.8**	**-3.8**	**-1.8**	0.2	0.2	0.2	**-3.8**	0.2	**-3.8**	**-3.8**	**-1.8**	**-1.8**	0.2	0.2	0.2	0.2	0.2	0.2	0.1 (0.5)
Gross Motor Coordination*	**-2**	**-7**	-0.8	0.5	-0.8	-0.8	**-3.3**	-0.8	-0.8	**-2**	**-3.3**	**-2**	0.5	0.5	**-4.5**	0.5	-0.8	**-2**	0.4 (0.8)
Fine Motor Coordination*	**-5.5**	**-2.4**	-1.6	-0.1	0.7	-0.8	**-3.2**	-1.6	**-3.9**	-1.6	-1.6	-0.8	-0.1	**-3.9**	**-3.9**	0.7	-1.6	-1.6	0.9 (1.3)
DCD Total*	**-5.3**	**-5.3**	**-1.8**	0.3	0.3	-0.8	**-4.3**	-1.3	**-3.8**	**-2.8**	**-2.8**	**-1.8**	0.3	**-2.3**	**-4.3**	0.8	-1.3	**-1.8**	1.5 (2.0)

Note: SS - Standard Score; Qualitative descriptions of IQ SS, percentage included in bell-shaped distribution are given in parenthesis : ≥ 130 (2.2%) = Very Superior, 120-129 (6.7%) = Superior, 110-119 (16.1%) = High Average, 90-109 (50%) = Average, 80-89 (16.1%) = Low Average, 70-79 (6.7%) = Borderline, ≤ 69 (2.2%) = Extremely Low; @ T-scores with Mean = 50; SD = 10, scores from 66 to 70 – much above average, scores>70 – very much above average, D = ADHD Index, A = Inattention, B = Hyperactivity/Impulsivity;* denotes z-score (relative to the control group used in this study); deviant scores (≤ -1.65) are marked in bold; z-scores used as covariates in the fMRI analysis are underlined. No participants with an FSIQ lower than the average score (90) were included in the study. As a result of this cut-off procedure, there were two DPs (DP14 and DP17) who had a VIQ lower than 90. Because the core deficits in dyslexia are in the language domain (Hulme and Snowling, 2009), scores on VIQ may be significantly lower in adult DPs than in the control group (Ramus et al., 2003).

These findings are in line with previous reports on spelling (Bruck, 1990; Hanley, 1997; Rack, 1997; Reid et al., 2007) and pseudoword reading in DPs (Bruck, 1990; Reid et al., 2007). Seventy two percent (13 DPs) and 66.7% (12 DPs) exhibited deficits on real word reading and irregular word reading, respectively. Two DPs (11.1%), including DP5 who had an FSIQ score within the superior range, did not show any deficit on any literacy measures, despite the fact that they were diagnosed with dyslexia (two years before being tested in this study) and explained in the interview that they had been suffering from literacy problems since starting school.

Table 3. Performance of individual DPs on literacy tests, pseudoword and irregular words reading tests

Measures/ Participant number	1	2	3	4	5	6	7	8	9	10	11	12	13	14	15	16	17	18	Controls
TOWRE Word Correct*	-1.3	**-6.5**	**-5.1**	**-3.1**	0.7	0.7	**-7.5**	**-2.3**	**-8.1**	**-4.7**	-0.9	**-4.9**	**-4.7**	**-4.5**	**-10.3**	**-4.3**	**-4.7**	-1.5	95.3 (5.0)
WRAT Spelling (% correct)*	-0.6	**-5.6**	**-4.4**	**-3.1**	-0.6	**-3.8**	**-2.5**	**-6.3**	**-5.0**	**-11.9**	**-3.8**	**-6.3**	**-1.9**	**-6.9**	**-12.5**	**-5.0**	**-5.0**	**-3.8**	80.0 (4.0)
TOWRE Pseudoword Correct*	0.2	**-3.8**	**-5.6**	**-4.4**	0.0	-1.0	**-3.0**	**-5.6**	**-5.2**	**-7.8**	**-3.2**	**-6.0**	**-5.2**	**-2.0**	**-8.2**	**-3.6**	**-7.0**	**-3.8**	57.1 (5.0)
Pseudoword (Coltheart) % correct*	1.0	-0.3	-0.7	-1.6	0.7	-0.3	-0.3	-0.3	-1.6	**-5.2**	0.0	**-2.6**	-1.6	0.3	**-1.9**	0.0	**-6.2**	**-2.3**	90.0 (10.2)
Pseudoword (Coltheart) Time (s)*	0.5	**-3.4**	**-8.2**	-1.1	0.3	-0.7	**-1.8**	**-3.1**	**-6.6**	**-17.3**	**-4.3**	**-8.2**	**-10.2**	**-2.3**	**-22.8**	**-4.5**	**-12.9**	**-2.9**	23.1 (4.4)
Pseudoword Reading Composite	0.8	**-3.6**	**-6.9**	**-3.4**	0.4	-1.0	**-2.4**	**-4.3**	**-6.4**	**-14.4**	**-3.6**	**-8.0**	**-8.1**	**-1.9**	**-15.7**	**-3.9**	**-12.5**	**-4.3**	88.5 (6.3)
Irregular word reading (% correct)*	1.3	-0.3	-0.8	-1.3	1.8	-0.3	0.8	**-4.2**	1.3	-1.3	-0.3	-0.3	-1.3	**-4.0**	-1.0	-1.3	**-2.4**	-1.3	18.9 (2.9)
Irregular word reading (time in sec.)*	-0.4	**-5.6**	**-13.8**	**-2.1**	-0.7	-0.7	-0.7	**-6.6**	**-8.0**	-1.4	0.0	**-4.5**	**-5.2**	**-4.2**	**-13.6**	**-5.6**	**-4.9**	**-1.8**	95.3 (5.0)
Irregular Word Reading Composite	0.5	**-3.2**	**-8.1**	**-1.9**	0.6	-0.6	0	**-6**	**-3.7**	-1.5	-0.2	**-2.7**	**-3.6**	**-4.5**	**-8.1**	**-3.8**	**-4**	**-1.7**	80.0 (4.0)

Note: *denotes z-score (relative to the control group used in this study); deviant scores ($\leq$ - 1.65) are marked in bold; the names of the composite measures are in Italics; SDs given in parentheses.

These indicate that either they were well compensated, at least as far as the behavioural measures were concerned, or that the commonly used measures of literacy used here are not sensitive enough to detect their deficit. Phonological awareness and phonological fluency are usually both treated as indices of phonological processing (Ramus and Szenkovits, 2008; Reid et al., 2007). If both measures are combined, then sixteen DPs (88.9%) in the sample, tested in this study, exhibited this deficit.

This is similar to the findings of Reid et al. (2007), where 86.7% of DPs had a phonological deficit, but different to Ramus et al.'s (2003) results, where 100% of DPs showed this impairment and to White et al.'s (2006) findings, where only 52.2% of DPs had this disorder (when defined as performance ≤ 1.65 below the mean of the CPs).One must be cautious, however, when making a comparison with the results reported by White et al. (2006), as they refer to child DPs.

Table 4. Performance of individual DPs on phonological awareness, phonological fluency and orthography measures

Measures/ Participant Number	1	2	3	4	5	6	7	8	9	10	11	12	13	14	15	16	17	18	CPs
Spoonerisms (time in secs)*	-0.3	**-3.8**	-0.1	-0.7	1.1	**-5.1**	-0.1	**-3.9**	**-5.4**	**-12.0**	**-5.9**	**-5.6**	**-1.9**	**-2.7**	**-3.4**	**-3.1**	**-4.0**	**-2.6**	81.3 (22.1)
Spoonerisms (% correct)*	-0.2	**-5.0**	-0.2	**-5.0**	1.0	**-5.0**	1.0	**-8.6**	-0.2	**-5.0**	**-7.4**	**-5.0**	**-2.6**	**-6.2**	-0.2	-1.4	**-3.8**	**-7.4**	93.2 (7.0)
Phonological Pseudoword Forced-Choice (mean RT in msec)*	-1.0	0.2	**-1.8**	-0.6	-0.2	**-3.0**	0.8	**-4.2**	**-5.5**	**-6.9**	**-3.7**	**-2.0**	-1.4	0.0	-0.5	0.3	2.7	-0.7	2973.2 (492.7)
Phonological Pseudoword Forced-Choice (% correct)*	0.4	0.4	-0.2	-1.1	0.7	1.1	-0.2	**-1.7**	-0.9	**-1.7**	**-1.8**	**-1.7**	0.0	**-2.0**	**-4.4**	**-2.9**	**-5.5**	**-3.3**	86.8 (9.1)
Phonological Awareness Composite	-0.5	**-3.4**	-1	**-3.1**	1.1	**-5**	0.6	**-7.6**	**-5**	**-10.6**	**-7.9**	**-5.9**	**-2.5**	**-4.5**	**-3.6**	**-3**	**-4.4**	**-5.8**	n/a
RAN Colour*	0.7	-0.1	-1.0	**-2.1**	0.5	0.2	**-2.3**	**-4.6**	-1.2	-1.2	-1.2	-0.4	-0.7	-1.5	**-3.7**	-0.7	-1.2	**-2.1**	34.4 (6.4)
RAN Picture*	0.8	0.2	-1.4	**-1.7**	0.5	-0.1	**-2.6**	**-4.0**	**-2.9**	-1.6	-0.5	-0.7	0.5	-1.3	**-4.9**	**-2.5**	-1.1	**-1.7**	39.4 (6.7)
RAN Digit*	0.3	**-2.3**	**-3.5**	**-2.7**	0.7	1.5	-1.4	-1.4	**-3.1**	**-5.2**	-0.6	-0.6	**-2.7**	-1.4	**-13.1**	-1.0	**-1.8**	**-1.8**	22.6 (2.4)
RAN Letter*	-0.4	**-2.1**	**-2.7**	**-1.4**	**-1.7**	-0.1	-1.4	-1.1	**-4.7**	**-8.7**	-0.4	**-1.7**	**-2.4**	**-1.7**	**-7.7**	-1.1	**-3.1**	**-1.7**	23.8 (3.0)
Phonological Fluency Composite	0.4	-1.3	**-2.7**	**-2.5**	0	0.5	**-2.4**	**-3.5**	**-3.7**	**-5.2**	-0.8	-1.1	-1.6	**-1.9**	**-9.2**	-1.6	**-2.3**	**-2.3**	n/a
Orthographic Word-Pseudo-homophone Choice (% correct)*	1.3	0.0	1.3	0.0	1.3	-0.4	-0.9	0.4	**-2.2**	**-4.5**	0.9	0.0	-0.9	-0.9	**-7.1**	**-4.0**	**-2.7**	0.0	95.0 (2.8)
Orthographic Word-Pseudo-homophone Choice test (mean RT in msec)*	-0.1	**-2.8**	**-1.8**	0.3	0.5	**-4.6**	0.2	**-1.7**	**-2.9**	**-3.6**	-0.9	-1.2	-1.1	**-6.7**	**-7.8**	**-1.8**	-0.1	-1.3	850.5 (163.7)
Orthography Composite	1.0	**-2.4**	-0.4	0.2	1.5	**-4.2**	-0.6	-1.0	**-4.2**	**-6.7**	0.0	-1.0	-1.6	**-6.3**	**-12.5**	**-4.8**	**-2.4**	-1.0	n/a

Note: *z-score (relative to the control group used in this study); deviant scores (≤ - 1.65) are marked in bold; the names of the composite measures are in Italics. SDs given in parentheses.

Eight DPs exhibited a deficit on the orthography composite based on the task, which although it involves phonological processing, biases towards orthographic processing through the stimulus design. One cannot decide which item: *'rane'* or *'rain'* is a real English word, on the basis of phonological form because it is the same for both items. One needs to access their orthographic lexicon to make this decision.

Summing up, the multiple case analysis of DPs' performance on psychometric tests revealed marked heterogeneity among DPs and this is in line with the previous findings (e.g., Ramus et al., 2003; Reid et al., 2007; White et al., 2006).

3.2. The fMRI Results

The neuroimaging results are shown in Figure 1 (please see also Appendix B Tables 1-18). The contrast CPs>DP show brain areas which were hypoactivated (underactivated) by a given individual DP, as compared to the control group, during word reading, relative to a control condition. Hypoactivation in functional neuroimaging studies is usually assumed to reflect a functional disruption in a system (Shaywitz et al., 1998). In the context of the main theories of dyslexia, which assume deficits in particular brain areas, hypoactivation (underactivation) in these areas is interpreted as lending support for these theories. The contrast DP>CPs reveals brain areas which were hyperactivated (overactivated) by a given individual DP, as compared to the control group, during word reading, relative to fixating on a cross. Hyperactivation in the functional neuroimaging studies is usually interpreted as a correlate of a compensatory mechanism (Brunswick et al., 1999; Pugh, Mencl, Shaywitz et al., 2000; Shaywitz et al., 1998). Because the main theories of dyslexia are concerned with a deficit and not compensatory mechanisms, hyperactivation (overactivation) of the brain areas associated with these main theories is not interpreted as evidence of support for them.

3.2.1. Neuroimaging Results for Individual DPs

It is important to emphasise that the neuroimaging results are not confounded by ADHD or DCD, because ADHD and DCD scores were used as covariates in the neuroimaging analyses. Furthermore, the neuroimaging results are not confounded by the BOLD response due to the 'button press' and 'Star' stimulus (used to monitor participants' vigilance in the scanner) because they were included in the design matrix as regressors. Finally, they are not confounded by differences in IQ (FSIQ), age or handedness between an individual DP and CPs as the scores for these variables were included in the fMRI analysis as covariates.

An inspection of Figure 1 and Appendix B Tables 1–18 reveals that individuals with dyslexia exhibited heterogeneous and complex patterns of hypoactivation which involved the areas predicted by the three main current theories of dyslexia. The results for every individual DP are presented below in the context of the predictions made by the main theories. The activation of every DP is compared to the activation of the CPs (treated as a group) because the focus of this chapter is on the individual differences among DPs.

DP1 exhibited underactivation in eight areas predicted by the PDT (L Area 6, L Area 44, L TE3, L IPC (PF), L IPC (PFcm), L IPC (PGp), L fusiform gyrus and L middle temporal gyrus). There was underactivation in one area postulated by the MDT (R hOC5 (V5)). DP1 showed underactivation in three areas hypothesised by the CDT (R Lobule VIIa Crus I (Hem), L Lobule VIIa Crus II (Hem) and R Lobule VIIa Crus II (Hem)). DP1 did not overactivate any areas associated with the three theories. Please see Figure 1 and Appendix B Table 1.

DP2 showed hypoactivation in three areas predicted by the CDT (L Lobule VIIa Crus I (Hem), R Lobule VIIa Crus I (Hem) and R Lobule VIIa Crus II (Hem)). The hypoactivation in L IPC (PF), predicted by the PDT, did not survive correction for the number of voxels (k<6). However, when the significance threshold was dropped to p<0.001 (uncorrected for the multiple comparisons), DP2 exhibited significant underactivation in L IPC (PF). (Because these thresholds are somewhat arbitrary, they could turn out to be too conservative and could mask a real effect, especially where heterogeneous populations (with respect to fMRI and behavioural profiles) are involved.

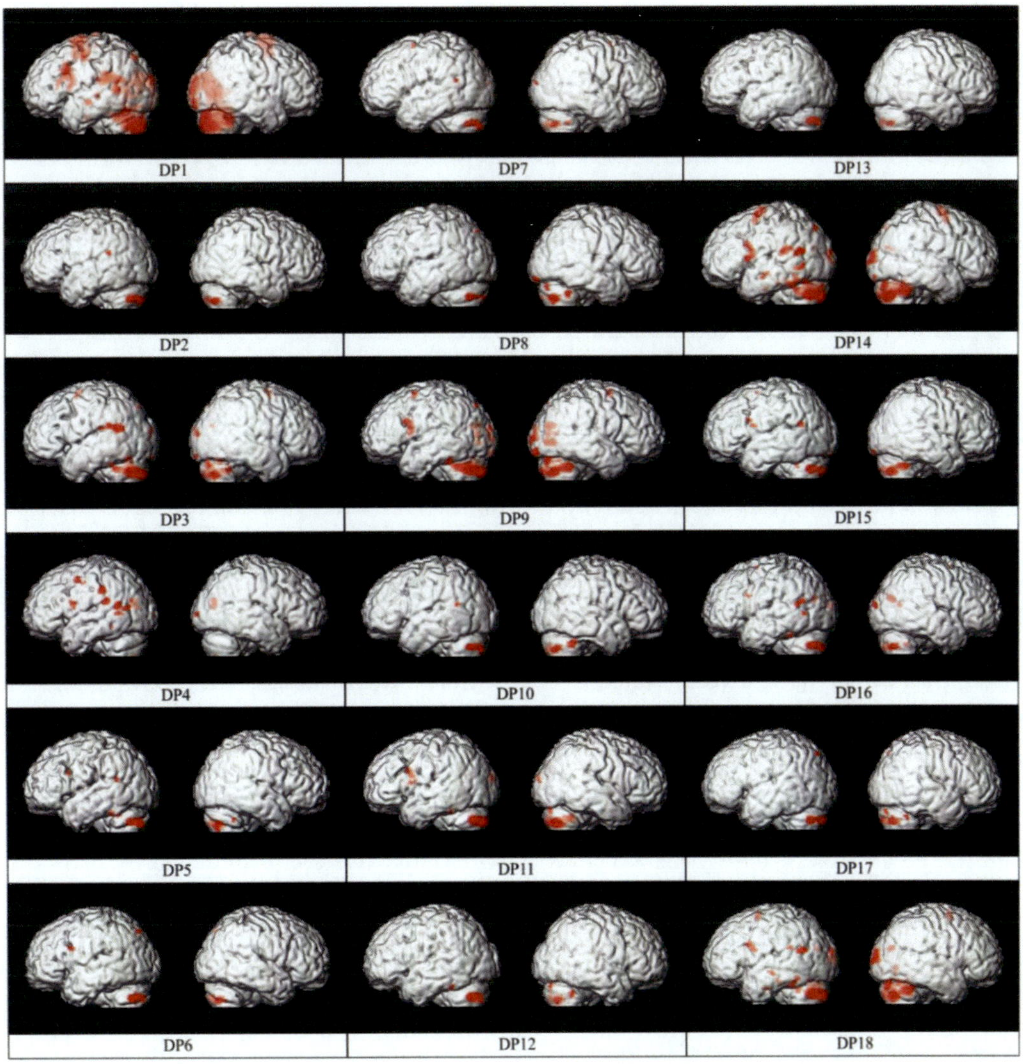

Figure 1. Clusters of underactivation (CPs>DP) for individual DPs. The results for DP1, DP3, DP6, DP9, DP10, DP11, DP12, DP14, DP15, DP16 and DP18 are at p<.05 FDR; the results for DP2, DP4, DP5, DP7, DP8, DP13 and DP17 are at p<.001 (uncorrected for multiple comparisons). Underactivation is superimposed on a volume rendered brain (a spatially normalised anatomical image for an individual DP). Cluster size threshold k≥6. An ROI mask was applied as described in the Method section.

Therefore it is of value to lower them in some cases to ascertain whether there is an effect at a lower threshold). There was no hypoactivation in the areas predicted by the MDT. DP2 did not exhibit any overactivation in the areas associated with the theories. Please see Figure 1 and Appendix B Table 2.

DP3 showed underactivation of some areas predicted by: the PDT (L Area 6, L Area 44, L Area 45, L middle temporal gyrus, L IPC (PF), L IPC (PFm), L IPC (PGp)), the MDT (R Area 17, L Area 18 and R Area 18) and the CDT (L Lobule VIIa Crus I (Hem), R Lobule VIIa Crus I (Hem) and R Lobule VIIa Crus II (Hem)). No overactivation was exhibited by DP3 in the areas associated with the theories. Please see Figure 1 and Appendix B Table 3.

DP4 exhibited no hypoactivation when the results were corrected for multiple comparisons. However, when the significance was lowered to $p<0.001$, uncorrected for multiple comparisons, DP4 showed hypoactivation in areas hypothesised by the PDT (L Area 6, L Area 44, L middle temporal gyrus, L fusiform gyrus, L TE3, L IPC (PF) and L IPC (PGp)), by the MDT (R Area 18) and by the CDT (L Lobule VIIb (Hem)) (please see Figure 1 and Table 4a in Appendix B). DP4 exhibited overactivation (FDR, $p<0.05$) in areas associated with the PDT (L Area 6, L Insula (Ig2), L IPC (PFm) and L IPC (PGa)), MDT (L Area 17, R Area 17, L Area 18 and R Area 18) and CDT (R Lobule VIIa Crus I (Hem), and L Lobule VI (Hem)). Please see Appendix B Table 4b.

DP5 showed underactivation in four areas predicted by the CDT (L Lobule VIIa Crus I (Hem), R Lobule VIIa Crus I (Hem), R Lobule VIIa Crus II (Hem) and R Lobule VI (Hem)). DP5 exhibited hypoactivation in one area predicted by the PDT (L Area 44), but it did not survive correction for the number of voxels ($k<6$). However, when the significance threshold was dropped to $p<0.001$ (uncorrected for the multiple comparisons), DP5 exhibited significant underactivation in L Area 44 and in L IPC (PFm). There was no underactivation in areas predicted by the visual MDT. DP5 overactivated ($p<0.001$, uncorrected for multiple comparisons) two areas associated with the visual MDT (L Area 17 and R Area 18). Please see Figure 1 and Appendix B Table 5.

DP6 showed underactivation in two areas predicted by the PDT (L Area 44 and L IPC (PGp)). DP6 also showed underactivation in three areas predicted by the CDT (L Lobule VIIa Crus I (Hem), R Lobule VIIa Crus I (Hem) and R Lobule VIIa Crus II (Hem)). There was no underactivation in the areas predicted by the MDT. DP6 did not overactivate any areas associated with the theories. Please see Figure 1 and Appendix B Table 6.

DP7 exhibited no underactivation in the areas predicted by any of the theories. However, when the significance threshold was lowered ($p<0.001$, uncorrected for multiple comparisons), he underactivated two areas predicted by the PDT (L Area 6 and L IPC (PFm)), one area predicted by the MDT (R Area 18) and five areas predicted by the CDT (L Lobule VIIa Crus I (Hem), R Lobule VIIa Crus I (Hem), L Lobule VIIa Crus II (Hem), R Lobule VIIa Crus II (Hem) and R Lobule VI (Hem)). There was no underactivation in the areas predicted by the MDT. No overactivation was exhibited by DP7 in the areas associated with the theories. Please see Figure 1 and Appendix B Table 7.

DP8 underactivated exclusively three areas predicted by the CDT (L Lobule VIIa Crus I (Hem), R Lobule VIIa Crus I (Hem) and R Lobule VIIa Crus II (Hem)). However, when the significance threshold was lowered to $p<0.001$ (uncorrected for multiple comparisons), DP8 underactivated one area predicted by the PDT (IPC (PGp)), two areas predicted by the MDT (R Area 18 and R Area 17) and one additional area predicted by the CDT (R Lobule VI (Hem)). DP8 overactivated ($p<0.001$, uncorrected for multiple comparisons) one area associated with the PDT (L Insula (Id1)) and one area associated with the MDT (L Area 18). Please see Figure 1 and Appendix B Table 8. DP8's profile will also be discussed later in the section 'Supplementary results (and discussion) for DP8 and DP15 who were possibly 'at risk' of DCD' below.

DP9 underactivated three areas predicted by the PDT (L Area 6, L Area 44 and L IPC(PGp)), four areas predicted by the MDT (L Area 17, R Area 17, L Area 18 and R Area 18) and four areas predicted by the CDT (L Lobule VIIa Crus I (Hem), R Lobule VIIa Crus I (Hem), R Lobule VIIa Crus II (Hem) and R Lobule VI (Hem)). DP9 did not overactivate any areas associated with the theories. Please see Figure 1 and Appendix B Table 9.

DP10 underactivated one area predicted by the PDT (L IPC (PFm)) and four areas predicted by the CDT (L Lobule VIIa Crus I (Hem), R Lobule VIIa Crus I (Hem), R Lobule VIIa Crus II (Hem) and R Lobule VI (Hem)). There was no hypoactivation in the areas predicted by the MDT. DP10 did not exhibit overactivation in any areas associated with the theories. Please see Figure 1 and Appendix B Table 10.

DP11 showed underactivation in L Area 44 and in L fusiform gyrus, as predicted by the PDT. There was also underactivation in two areas predicted by the MDT (L Area 18 and R Area 18). Finally, DP11 exhibited underactivation in five areas predicted by the CDT (L Lobule VIIa Crus I (Hem), R Lobule VIIa Crus I (Hem), L Lobule VIIa Crus II (Hem), R Lobule VIIa Crus II (Hem) and R Lobule VI (Hem)). There was no overactivation in the areas associated with the theories. Please see Figure 1 and Appendix B Table 11.

DP12 underactivated one area predicted by the PDT (L fusiform gyrus) and five areas predicted by the CDT (L Lobule VIIa Crus I (Hem), R Lobule VIIa Crus I (Hem), L Lobule VIIa Crus II (Hem), R Lobule VIIa Crus II (Hem) and R Lobule VI (Hem)). DP12 did not underactivate any areas predicted by the MDT. There was no overaction in any areas associated with the theories. Please see Figure 1 and Appendix B Table 12.

DP13 exhibited no underactivation in the areas predicted by any of the theories. However, when the significance threshold was lowered ($p<0.001$, uncorrected for multiple comparisons), she exhibited hypoactivation in three areas predicted by the CDT (L Lobule VIIa Crus I (Hem), R Lobule VIIa Crus I (Hem) and R Lobule VIIa Crus II (Hem)). There was no underactivation in the areas predicted by the PDT and MDT. DP13 show overactivation ($p<0.001$, uncorrected for multiple comparisons) in two areas associated with the PDT (L Area 6 and L middle temporal gyrus) and one area associated with the MDT (L Area 17). Please see Figure 1 and Appendix B Table 13.

DP14 exhibited underactivation in seven areas predicted by the PDT (L Area 6, L Area 44, L middle temporal gyrus, L TE 3, L IPC (PFm), L IPC (PF) and L IPC (PGp)) two areas predicted by the MDT (L Area 18 and R Area 18) and five areas predicted by the CDT (L Lobule VIIa Crus I (Hem), R Lobule VIIa Crus I (Hem), R Lobule VIIa Crus II (Hem), R Lobule VI (Hem) and R Lobule VI (Vermis)). DP14 did not overactivate any areas associated with the theories. Please see Figure 1 and Appendix B Table 14.

DP15 underactivated four areas predicted by the PDT (L Area 6, L Area 44, L IPC (PGa) and L IPC (PGp)), one area predicted d by the MDT (R Area 17) and four areas predicted by the CDT (L Lobule VIIa Crus I (Hem), R Lobule VIIa Crus I (Hem), R Lobule VIIa Crus II (Hem) and L Lobule VI (Hem)). DP15 did not show overactivation in any areas associated with the theories. Please see Figure 1 and Appendix B Table 15. DP15's profile will also be discussed later in the section 'Supplementary results (and discussion) for DP8 and DP15 who were possibly 'at risk' of DCD' below.

DP16 exhibited hypoactivation in five areas predicted by the PDT (L Area 6, L Area 44, L middle temporal gyrus, L fusiform gyrus and L IPC (PFm)), one area predicted by the MDT (R Area 18) and four areas predicted by the CDT (L Lobule VIIa Crus I (Hem), R Lobule VIIa Crus I (Hem), R Lobule VIIa Crus II (Hem) and R Lobule VI (Hem)). There was no overactivation in any areas associated with the theories. Please see Figure 1 and Appendix B Table 16.

DP17 showed underactivation in three areas predicted by the CDT (L Lobule VIIa Crus I (Hem), R Lobule VIIa Crus I (Hem) and L Lobule VIIa Crus II (Hem)). There was no underactivation in the areas predicted by the MDT. DP17 exhibited underactivation in one area predicted by the PDT (L IPC (PGp)), but it did not survive correction for the number of voxels ($k<6$). However, when the significance threshold was dropped to $p<0.001$ (uncorrected for the multiple comparisons), DP17 exhibited significant underactivation in L IPC (PGp) and in and R Lobule VIIa Crus II (Hem). There was no hypoactivation in the areas predicted by the MDT. DP17 exhibited overactivation ($p<0.001$, uncorrected for multiple comparisons) in two areas associated with the PDT (L fusiform gyrus and L Insula (Id1)) and one area associated with the CDT (L Lobule VIIb (Hem)). Please see Figure 1 and Appendix B Table 17.

DP18 underactivated seven areas predicted by the PDT (L Area 6, L Area 44, L middle temporal gyrus, L fusiform gyrus, L TE 3, L IPC (PF) and L IPC (PFm)), two areas predicted by the MDT (L Area 18 and R Area 18) and four areas predicted by the CDT (L Lobule VIIa Crus I (Hem), R Lobule VIIa Crus I (Hem), R Lobule VIIa Crus II (Hem), and L Lobule VI (Hem)). DP18 did not overactivate any areas associated with the theories. Please see Figure 1 and Appendix B Table 18.

3.2.1.1. Supplementary Results (and Discussion) for DP8 and DP15 Who Were Possibly 'at Risk' of DCD

DP8 and DP15 were identified in this study as possibly being 'at risk' of DCD, therefore their neuroimaging results were also analysed for potential underactivation (and overactivation) (as compared to the CPs) in the areas which have been reported to be underactivated in participants with DCD. However, it needs to be born in mind that similar to developmental dyslexia, there is no consensus regarding the underlying cause of DCD. Furthermore, it needs to be stressed that the BOLD signal in this study is from a reading task, and not from a task that is typically used to investigate DCD.

It was reported (Kashiwagi, Iwaki, Narumi, Tamai, and Suzuki, 2009) that participants with DCD (in comparison to CPs) exhibited significantly lower brain activation in the L posterior parietal cortex and L postcentral gyrus during a visuo-motor task. The authors concluded that the dysfunction of these areas could be the neural underpinnings of a deficit of motor skill in participants with DCD. The coordinates with significant differences between the groups, reported by Kashiwagi et al. (2009) labeled by the AT V.1.8 (Eickhoff et al., 2005), had the following labels, probabilities and ranges: [MNI: x=-40, y=-48, z=66 – L SPL (7PC), probability=10%, range=0-20%; [MNI: x=-36, y=-52, z=50 – assigned to L hIP3 (probability=30%, range=10-40%), other overlapping areas: L SPL (7A), (probability=30%, range=20-40%), L hIP1 (probability=20%, range=0-30%), SPL (7PC) (probability=10%, range=10-50)]. The following MNI coordinates reported by Kashiwagi et al. (2009) x=-68, y=-20, z= 34 were not found in any probability map in the AT V.1.8. For clarity these areas are briefly described below. An observer-independent cytoarchitectonic mapping of the superior parietal cortex in 10 human postmortem brains of BA7 (Scheperjans, Eickhoff et al., 2008; Scheperjans, Hermann et al., 2008) showed that there are four areas within BA7. 7PC and 7A are two out of these four areas. Area 7PC is located on the lateral aspect of the anterior superior parietal lobule, posterior to BA2, and lateral to area 5L (an area within BA5, located in the postcentral sulcus near to the interhemispheric fissure). Area 7A, on the other hand, occupies the largest part of the superior parietal lobule and extends onto the precuneus and into the medial wall of the intraparietal sulcus. Cytoarchitectonic identification and probabilistic mapping was used to delineate hIP1 (human intraparietal area 1) (Choi et al., 2006). This area is located posterior and medial to human intraparietal area 2 (hIP2) and it is always within the depths of the intraparietal sulcus (Choi et al., 2006). Finally, hIP3 (human intraparietal area 3) is delineated in the anterior medial wall of the intraparietal sulcus (Scheperjans, Eickhoff et al., 2008; Scheperjans, Hermann et al., 2008).

There is now growing evidence that DCD may be associated with an impaired cerebellum (Brookes, Nicolson, and Fawcett, 2007; Ivry, 2003; Marien, Wackenier, De Surgeloose, De Deyn, and Verhoeven, 2010; O'Hare and Khalid, 2002). Furthermore, there is also evidence from animal models (Gramsbergen, 2003) which supports this hypothesis. As DCD is defined as a marked impairment in the development of motor coordination, the peak coordinates and cerebellar lobules of the significant ALE maxima for the meta-analysis for the experiments involving motor tasks (Stoodley and Schmahmann, 2009) were extracted. These coordinates were labeled with the AT V.1.8 (Eickhoff et al., 2005) and had the following labels, probabilities and ranges: [MNI: x=22, y=-56 z=-28 – R Lobule VI (Hem), probability=67%, range=67-94%; MNI: x=12, y=-64, z=-46 – R Lobule VIIIb (Hem), probability=42%, range=36-68% and R Lobule IX (Hem), probability=40%, range=1-46%; MNI: x=30, y=-66, z=-56 – R Lobule VIIb (Hem), probability=61%, range=30-61% and R Lobule VIIIa (Hem) probability=33%, range=33-68%; MNI: x=6, y=-64, z=-10 – R Lobule V, probability=49%, range=5-49].

A ROI mask with ten areas (*L SPL (7PC), L SPL (7A), L hIP1, L hIP3, R Lobule VI (Hem), R Lobule VIIIb (Hem), R Lobule IX (Hem), R Lobule VIIb (Hem), R Lobule VIIIa (Hem)* and *R Lobule V (Hem and Vermis)*) has been constructed using the AT V.1.8 (create composite option). The second level analysis (unpaired t-test) using SPM5 involved the following contrasts CPs>DP and DP>CPs, for DP8 and DP15. The analysis was the same as for the main results presented in this chapter with two exceptions: 1) a different mask was used as described above and 2) no 'DCD Total' variable was used as a covariate; this is because the aim of the analysis was to test whether DP8 and DP15 exhibited (in comparison with the CPs) any significant underactivation (or overactivation) in areas associated with DCD. The results are reported at $p<0.05$ FDR. The results for DP8 revealed significant underactivation in one parietal area (L hIP1) and three cerebellar areas (R Lobule V (Vermis), R Lobule VI (Hem) and R Lobule VIIb (Hem)). Interestingly, DP8 also exhibited overactivation in one parietal area (L SPL (7A)) and two cerebellar areas (R Lobule VIIIb (Hem) and R Lobule IX (Hem)) (please see Appendix C Table 1). DP15 showed underactivation in one parietal area (L SPL (7A)) and three cerebellar areas (R Lobule V (Vermis), R Lobule V (Hem) and R Lobule VI (Hem)). He did not exhibit any overactivation (please see Appendix C Table 2). Different profiles of underactivation (and overactivation) in these two DPs underscores the issue of individual differences in DCD.

The intriguing question arises of how to observe the effects of underactivation in DP8 and DP15 in the areas associated with movement during a reading task. This question becomes slightly less intriguing if one appreciates that: 1) a recent study reported by Heim et al. (2012) showed that L SPL (7A) is most likely involved in the general aspects of motor sequencing, including the sequencing of speech; 2) hIP1 (and hIP3) has been observed (Gillebert, Mantini, Peeters, Dupont, and Vandenberghe, 2013), using resting-state fMRI, to be highly correlated with R IPC (PFm) - an area homologous to L IPC (PFm) which, as described in the Introduction, is involved in phonological processing; 3) the R Lobule V (Hem) exhibits functional connectivity with the R Lobule VIIa Crus II (Hem); the R Lobule VIIb (Hem) shows functional connectivity with the L Lobule VI (Hem); R Lobule VI (Hem) exhibits functional connectivity with the L Lobule VIIa Crus II (Hem) (Bernard et al., 2012); all three lobules, with which the lobules underactivated in DP8 and DP15 exhibit functional connectivity, are involved in language processing (Stoodley and Schmahmann, 2009). It should be noted that R Lobule VI (Hem) was used in both masks (the ROI mask for the main study and the ROI for the 'DCD analysis' for DP8 and DP15). This is because this lobule was reported for both language tasks and motor tasks (Stoodley and Schmahmann, 2009). No DPs showed significant underactivation exclusively of this lobule in the main analysis.

Sumarising, the results suggest that both DP8 and DP15 exhibited a pattern of underactivation that seems to be consistent, in some aspects, with the patterns of underactivation observed in participants with DCD. DP8 additionally exhibited overactivation in one parietal area and two cerebellar areas hypothesised to be associated with DCD. This indicates that these areas can be used for compensatory mechanisms which are shaped on an individual basis. The results lend support to the claim that DP8 and DP15, who have only been diagnosed with dyslexia, additionally exhibit comorbid DCD.

4. Discussion

4.1. The Findings with Respect to the Main Theories of Dyslexia

The main goal of the research reported here was to investigate the neural correlates of reading deficit in dyslexia as predicted by the main theories of this disorder, with special emphasis on individual differences. The predictions of the main theories on the neural correlates of reading impairment in dyslexia were contrasted in the same individuals with dyslexia, as compared to the control group.

Underactivation in a given area (as specified in the Introduction) in a given individual DP was interpreted as support for a given theory of dyslexia. Additionally, overactivation was interpreted as activation in response to a deficit and as such consistent with a compensatory mechanism, as described in some earlier publications on dyslexia (Brunswick et al., 1999; Shaywitz et al., 1998).

If the reading deficit in DPs is due to phonological magnocellular or cerebellar impairments, as predicted by the PDT, MDT and CDT, respectively, then DPs should exhibit underactivation in comparison with CPs, in some or all areas within the phonological, visual magnocellular or cerebellar processing networks, specified in the Introduction.

Following these assumptions, the results, which involved underactivation in the areas postulated by the main theories, are summarised in Figure 2, below. The neural correlates of reading deficit in seventeen DPs (94.4% - all DPs except for DP13) were consistent with the predictions of the PDT and the CDT. The reading deficits of ten DPs (56%) - DP3, DP4, DP7, DP8, DP9, DP11, DP14, DP15, DP16 and DP18) were consistent with the predictions of the VDT, but not with the visual MDT. The reading deficit of DP13 was in agreement with only the CDT. Finally, the reading deficit of DP1 was consistent with all three theories of dyslexia (the PDT, visual MDT and CDT).

Summarising, the neural correlates of Word reading deficit are consistent with the PDT in seventeen cases (94.4%), with the CDT in eighteen cases (100%) and in one case (5.5%) with the MDT.

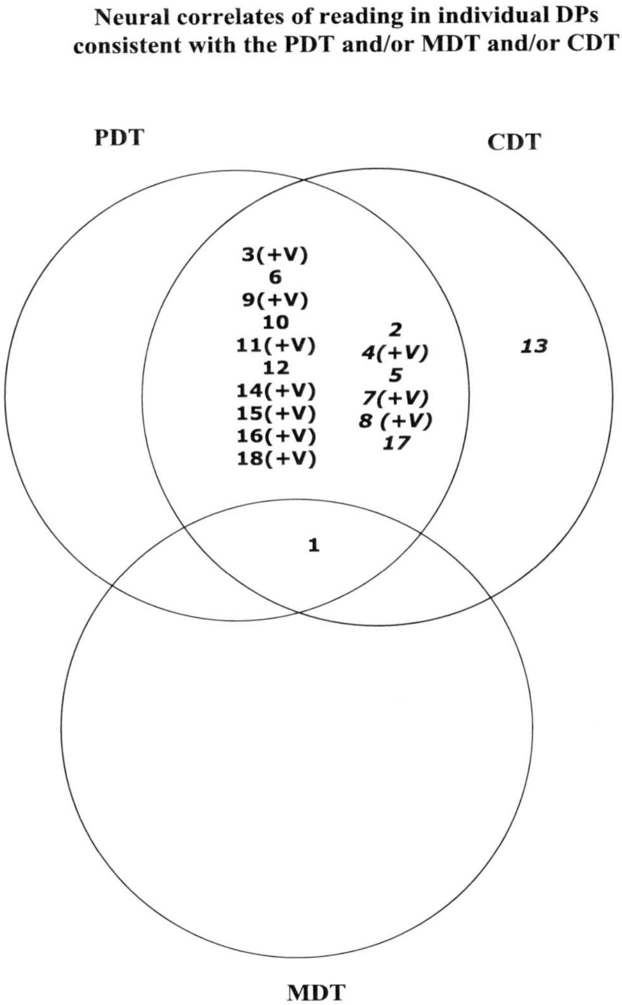

Figure 2. The distribution of individual DPs for whom reading impairment is consistent with the predictions of the PDT and/or MDT, and/or CDT, as revealed by the neuroimaging data (underactivation) of word reading. The numbers represent individual DPs. Underactivation for DPs (in regular typeface) is reported at p<0.05 FDR, hypoactivation for DPs (in Italics) is reported at p<0.001 (uncorrected for multiple comparisons). '+V' denotes that the neural correlates of reading impairment are not consistent with the predictions of the visual MDT, but the areas involved are consistent with the VDT.

The reading deficit of ten cases (56%) was consistent with the VDT, but not with the visual MDT, this is because in these cases, areas which receive input from both magno and parvo cells are underactivated, but not the V5/MT – the area which predominantly receives the magnocellular input.

Taking into consideration the additional predictions of the CDT, it is possible that the underactivation in phonological areas in all DPs (except DP13) is also consistent with the CDT (as well as with the PDT), but this holds only from the perspective of the CDT and not the perspective of the PDT. Finally, it is possible that the underactivation in phonological areas in DP1 is also in line with the predictions of the MDT, however, this is true only from the perspective of the visual MDT and not from the perspective of the PDT.

4.1.1. The Nature of the Neural Correlates of Reading Impairment in DPs in the Context of the Main Theories

4.1.1.1. The Phonological Deficit Theory

The data show that DPs have a heterogeneous pattern of underactivations in terms of localisation and extent – please see Appendix B Tables 1-18 for more details and Figures 1 and 2 for summaries). Focusing on localisation first, DPs with underactivation of the areas predicted by the PDT, exhibit hypoactivation in the anterior, temporal and posterior areas (DP1, DP3, DP4 DP16 and DP18), anterior and posterior areas (DP5, DP6, DP7 DP9 and DP15), and anterior and temporal areas (DP11).

Some DPs exhibited underactivation just within the posterior areas (DP2, DP8, DP10, and DP17), or temporal areas (DP12). The extent of the underactivations in individual DPs within the phonological areas ranged from small clusters (k=6 voxels), through medium (k=80 voxels) to relatively large clusters (k=528 voxels).

As discussed above, a number of neuroimaging studies have reported that DPs use frontal areas (L and R Areas 44, 45 and 6) for compensation (Brunswick et al., 1999; Pugh, Mencl, Shaywitz et al., 2000; Shaywitz et al., 1998), although as discussed earlier, a more recent meta-analysis (Maisog et al., 2008) revealed no support for hyperactivity in the L anterior areas in DPs, suggesting that neuroimaging results in these areas are likely to be more varied in their spatial location and their reproducibility. The claim that DPs tend to overactivate the anterior areas is supported here by two cases (DP4 and DP13) (11%).

As discussed earlier, Paulesu et al. (1996) put forward a hypothesis that the deficient phonological system of DPs is due to a dysfunctional L insula which acts as a connecting bridge between the anterior and posterior language areas. However, other researchers (e.g., Rumsey et al., 1997; Shaywitz et al., 1998) did not find evidence for a functionally impaired L insula in DPs. The study reported here found no support for underactivation of the L insula. In contrast, DP4 overactivated L Insula (Ig2), and DP8 and DP17 overactivated L Insula (Id1). Note, however, that the currently available cytoarchitectonic maps of the insula (Kurth et al., 2009) do not cover the entire insula.

As discussed in the Introduction, the neuroimaging studies, which compare a group of DPs and CPs, revealed that DPs, as a group, when reading, show underactivation relative to CPs in the L dorsal sub-system (angular gyrus, Wernicke's area and the supramarginal gyrus) and the L ventral sub-system (inferior occipito-temporal fusiform area) (e.g., Brunswick et al., 1999; Paulesu et al., 2001; Pugh, Mencl, Jenner et al., 2000; Salmelin et al., 1996;

Shaywitz et al., 1998). First, the focus here is on the results which have a bearing on the L dorsal sub-system.

Eight DPs (DP1, DP4, DP6, DP8, DP9, DP14, DP15 and DP17) (44.4%) demonstrated underactivation of the L angular gyrus. DP15 underactivated both L IPC (PGa) and L IPC (PGp), the other seven DPs (38.9%) underactivated L IPC (PGp). However, DP4 showed overactivation of the L IPC (PGa). Regarding Wernicke's area, four DPs (DP1, DP4, DP14 and DP18) demonstrated underactivation in L Area TE3 (Caspers et al., 2008). Note, however, that there is currently no cytoarchitectonic map available of the entire Wernicke's area.

With respect to another dorsal area - BA40, six DPs (DP1, DP2, DP3, DP4, DP14, and DP18) showed underactivation in the L IPC (PF). Seven DPs (DP3, DP5, DP7, DP10, DP14, DP16 and DP18) demonstrated hypoactivation in the L IPC (PFm). DP1 also showed underactivation in L IPC (PFcm). No underactivation was noted in any DP for L IPC (PFop) and L IPC (PFt). Three DPs (DP11, DP12 and DP13) did not exhibit underactivation in BA40. One DP (DP4) overactivated L IPC (PFm).

The results from the current multiple-case study for the L dorsal sub-system show a picture that seems to be more complex than the one which emerged from the studies employing only group comparisons (DPs vs CPs). First, not all DPs exhibited underactivation in these areas. Second, DP4 exhibited overactivation in two areas within this system. Neither finding is congruent with the results reported for group comparisons involving adults with dyslexia compared with controls.

Focusing on the L ventral area (L BA37, L BA21 and VWFA), it was reported (Brunswick et al., 1999) that both during explicit and implicit reading, DPs exhibited reduced activation in the L BA37 relative to CPs. The authors suggested that because of BA37's involvement in modality-independent naming, the reduced activation in DPs can be interpreted as a neural correlate of impairment in lexical retrieval. The data from the experiment reported in this chapter show that six DPs (DP1, DP4, DP11, DP12, DP16 and DP18) demonstrated underactivation of the L fusiform gyrus. In contrast, DP17 exhibited overactivation of the L fusiform gyrus. However, there are currently no probabilistic cytoarchitectonic maps of L fusiform gyrus.

Regarding the L middle temporal gyrus (BA21), the data show that six DPs (DP1, DP3, DP4, DP14, DP16 and DP18) exhibited underactivation of this area. In contrast, DP13 exhibited overactivation in L middle temporal gyrus. Note that, as for BA37, there are no probabilistic cytoarchitectonic maps currently available of BA21.

Finally, as discussed in the Introduction, Cohen, Lehericy et al. (2002) put forward a hypothesis stating that visual word form representations: "are subtended by a restricted patch of the L hemispheric fusiform cortex [average Talairach coordinates x=-43, y=-54, z=-12] which is reproducibly activated by reading" (p. 1054). However, McCrory et al. (2005), on the basis of their research (please see Introduction) concluded that this area must be involved in a more general deficit in the binding of visual with phonological information. These Talairach coordinates were transformed here using Brett's (1999) formula which gave the following MNI coordinates: x=-43, y=-55, z=-17. No DP exhibited underactivation for these exact coordinates, however six DPs (DP1, DP4, DP11, DP12, DP16 and DP18) showed underactivation within a sphere of 15 mm around these coordinates (mean coordinates with SDs: x=-40.3 (2.4), y=-47.4 (10.4), z=-20.3 (6.4)) (please see Appendix B Tables 1, 4, 11, 12,

16 and 18 for details). One DP (DP17) overactivated an area in close proximilty to VWFA (the coordinates for the local maximum were x=-30, y=-52, z=-8).

Similar to the results for the L dorsal sub-system, the results for the L ventral sub-system from the current multiple-case study underscore the fact that the picture seems to be more complex than the one which has emerged from the studies based only on group comparisons (DPs vs CPs). First, not all DPs exhibited underactivation in the L dorsal sub-system, as one would predict from reported group studies. Second, two DPs showed overactivation in this subsystem. Both results are not in agreement with the outcomes of studies which reported only group comparisons.

4.1.1.2. The Cerebellar Deficit Theory

Heterogeneous patterns (in terms of localisation and extent) of underactivation among DPs were also noted in the areas associated with the CDT. The data presented here on cerebellar involvement in the neural correlates of reading deficit in DPs shows that there is support for functional abnormality in the R Lobule VIIa Crus I (Hem) in 94.4% of cases. However, DP4 showed overactivation in the R Lobule VIIa Crus I (Hem). This lobule was found to be functionally activated in language studies with CPs (Stoodley and Schmahmann, 2009), including silent reading (Fulbright et al., 1999). Functional abnormality in the L Lobule VIIa Crus I (Hem) was noted in sixteen cases (89%). Similar to its RH counterpart, this area was found to be activated in language processing (Stoodley and Schmahmann, 2009), including silent reading (Fulbright et al., 1999). Nine cases (50%) supported the claim that there is functional abnormality in the R Lobule VI (Hem). Two cases (11.1%) confirmed that there was functional abnormality in the L Lobule VI (Hem). The R and L Lobule VI (Hem) were found to be functionally activated in language tasks with CPs (Stoodley and Schmahmann, 2009). Five cases (28%) supported the claim that there is functional abnormality in L Lobule VIIa Crus II (Hem). Seventeen cases (94%) supported the claim of functional abnormality in DPs' R Lobule VIIa Crus II (Hem). There is support in one case (5.6%) for functional abnormality for the L Lobule VIIb (Hem). The L Lobule VIIb (Hem) has a representation of the whole body (Brodal, 1981) and within this lobule (and R Lobule VIIb (Hem)) the biggest significant difference was found between DPs' and CPs' brains in a histological study (Finch et al., 2002) (please see Introduction for details). DP17, however, overactivated L Lobule VIIb (Hem). Finally, one DP underactivated R Lobule VI (Vermis). This lobule was reported to be involved in language processing (Stoodley and Schmahmann, 2009). Furthermore, R Lobule VI (Vermis) (together with the R lentiform nucleus), as discussed above, was reported (Pernet et al., 2009) to differentiate DPs and CPs in such a way that 100% of DPs fell outside the 95% confidence interval boundaries of CPs. It was hypothesised (Pernet et al., 2009) that R Lobule VI (Vermis) is important for the automatisation of skills. If this hypothesis is true, then this result may indicate that DP14 exhibits deficits in automaticity during reading.

The data presented in this study did not record underactivation in any individual DP (relative to CPs) in the R Lobule VIIb (Hem) which (together with L Lobule VIIb (Hem), and L and R Lobule VIIa Crus II (Hem)) differentiated well between DPs' and CPs' (Finch et al., 2002).

The extent of underactivations in individual DPs within the cerebellar areas ranged from small clusters (k=6 voxels), through medium (k=51-98) and large (k=104-845) to relatively very large clusters (1168-5420).

Although the fMRI studies based on group comparisons (DPs and CPs) report mixed results (for instance please see the meta-analysis of functional neuroimaging studies of dyslexia by Maisog et al. (2008)), the multiple case study reported here showed support for the predictions of the CDT in all cases (100%). However, the results from the study reported here reveal a more complex picture than one could expect on the basis of the neuroimaging literature involving exclusively between group comparisons (DPs vs CPs). First, the pattern of underactivation in the cerebellum in DPs reported in this study shows heterogeneity. Second, two cases (11.1%) exhibited overactivation in the cerebellar areas hypothesised to exhibit underactivation by the CDT. As all DPs exhibited underactivation of the cerebellum, 100% of cases are consistent with cerebellar deficit. However, the results which involve overactivation suggest, in contrast to the predictions of the CDT, that some areas of the cerebellum in some DPs may be unimpaired and may be used for compensation.

One could ask the question why there is such heterogeneity in terms of the spatial localisation and extent of activations in the cerebellum in individual DPs. There may be at least two reasons for this. First, research shows that the cerebellum is one of the first brain structures to begin to differentiate, however it is one of the last brain structures to achieve maturity. This prolonged maturational process makes the cerebellum particularly susceptible to disruptions during the process of embryogenesis (Wang and Zoghbi, 2001).

Second, the cerebellum exhibits considerable plasticity (e.g., Black, Isaacs, Anderson, Alcantara, and Greenough 1990; Klintsova, Goodlett, and Greenough, 2000; Schlang, 2001; Zheng and Raman, 2010). These characteristics suggest that the cerebellum may be influenced by many different factors during the ontogenetic development of a DP (Bishop, 2002) and these may differ on individual basis.

Summarising, the current study provides one of the most detailed insights into the differences between cerebellar involvement in reading impairment in dyslexia in a multiple-case study.

4.1.1.3. The Magnocellular Deficit Theory

With regard to the MDT, the word reading deficit of one DP (5.5%) was consistent with the MDT. The MDT turned out to be the most difficult to evaluate. This is because only the L and R V5/MT is thought to receive input predominantly from the magnocellular stream (Tootell and Taylor, 1995; Watson et al., 1993) and this area is characterised by considerable variation between participants, in the extent and location of the standard space (Malikovic et al., 2007).

Furthermore, the effect in the V5/MT could have been weakened due to the image stabilization, needed also in the control condition (i.e. fixating on the '+') which was necessary in this study and considered to be a better overall control condition than the 'rest condition'. (This is because the 'rest' control condition provides an opportunity for the participants to 'daydream' or 'ruminate' which results in stimulus-independent thoughts (Binder et al., 1999), and because thoughts quite often have language content this could be a potential confound in the observed brain activation for an experiment which relies on a language based task). Nevertheless, the effect due to letter localization (needed in the experimental condition, but not in the control condition) should not have been weakened by the control condition and therefore should be detectible.

The other two areas R and L V1, and R and L V2 consist of partially separated magno and parvo cells (Wurtz and Kandel, 2000), therefore, underactivation in any of these areas may reflect underactivation of either magno cells, or parvo cells or a combination of the two. Hence, the approach taken in this chapter was to interpret underactivation in V1 and V2 as supporting the visual MDT, only if it was found jointly with underactivation in V5/MT.

In contrast, the underactivation in V1 and/or V2, in the absence of underactivation in V5/MT was interpreted as consistent with the predictions of a hypothetical Visual Deficit Theory (VDT), but not in line with the predictions the visual MDT. The results for ten DPs (56%) were consistent with the VDT, but not with the visual MDT.

4.1.2. The Neuroimaging Results for Individual DPs in the Context of Their Behavioural Scores for Word Reading

The neuroimaging and TOWRE results divide DPs into two subgroups. The first sub-group consists of thirteen DPs (DP2, DP3, DP4, DP7, DP8, DP9, DP10, DP12, DP13, DP14, DP15, DP16 and DP17) who showed a clear deficit on word reading (TOWRE) and also exhibited underactivation when reading words, as predicted by one of the main theories. Despite the reading test in the scanner probably being easier than TOWRE, the DPs in this sub-group exhibited underactivation.These DPs are not therefore compensated on the behavioural level, with respect to word reading, and this is clearly reflected on the neural level.

The second sub-group consists of five DPs (DP1, DP5, DP6, DP11 and DP18) who exhibited no word reading deficit on TOWRE (despite having a recent diagnosis of dyslexia and a history of literacy difficulties), but showed clear underactivation in the neuroimaging results on word reading, as predicted by at least one of the main theories. These DPs are clearly compensated on word reading on the behavioural level, however, the neuroimaging results uncovered a lack of compensation on the neural level, even on, the probably easier reading test than TOWRE, administered in the MRI scanner (please see Method section).

4.1.3. DPs' Neuroimaging Results in the Context of the Psychometric Summary and Composite Variables

Looking from the broader perspective of literacy, phonological and orthographic measures and neuroimaging results, one could ask whether DPs who have a similar profile on behavioural measures also have a similar profile on their neuroimaging results. As shown in Table 5 below, there are five subgroups of DPs who exhibited a similar profile on the behavioural measures. Subgroup 1 consists of: DP9, DP14, DP15 and DP17; DP4 and DP8 belong to Subgroup 2; Subgroup 3 consists of DP2 and DP16; DP12 and DP13 belong to Subgroup 4. Finally, DP1 and DP5 belong to Subgroup 5.

Putting the behavioural results for these subgroups in the context of the neuroimaging results for word reading, three out of the four DPs (DP9, DP14 and DP15) from Subgroup 1 exhibited similar patterns of neuroimaging results with the neural correlates of reading being consistent with the PDT, CDT and VDT. DP17 exhibited a different profile with neuroimaging results consistent with only the PDT and CDT.

The neural correlates of reading for DP4 and DP8 (Subgroup 2) differed because they were consistent with the predictions of the PDT and CDT in DP8, but with the predictions of the PDT, CDT and VDT in DP4. The neural correlates of reading in DP2 and DP16 from Subgroup 3 also differed because they were in agreement with the predictions of the PDT and CDT in DP2, but with the PDT, CDT and VDT in DP16. DP12 and DP13 (from Subgroup 4) exhibited different profiles on the neural level. Underactivation consistent with the PDT and CDT was exhibited by DP12, whereas the neural correlates of DP13's reading were consistent with only the CDT. Finally, subgroup 5 (DP1 and DP5) exhibited different profiles on the neuroimaging results. DP1 showed underactivation consistent with the predictions of all three main theories (the PDT, visual MDT and CDT), whereas DP5 showed underactivation consistent with the PDT and CDT.

Table 5. Neuroimaging results for individual DPs in the context of the psychometric summary variables

Measures / number of an individual DP	9	14	15	17	2	4	8	10	16	3	12	13	18	7	11	6	1	5
Behavioural measures/ number of deficits	7/7 deficits				6/7 deficits					5/7 deficits				4/7 deficits	3/7 deficits		0/7 deficits	
Literacy measures																		
TOWRE Word Correct*	X	X	X	X	X	X	X	X	X	X	X	X	+	X	+	+	+	+
Pseudoword Reading Composite	X	X	X	X	X	X	X	X	X	X	X	X	X	X	X	+	+	+
Irregular Word Reading Composite	X	X	X	X	X	X	X	+	X	X	X	X	X	+	+	+	+	+
WRAT Spelling (% correct)*	X	X	X	X	X	X	X	X	X	X	X	X	X	X	X	X	+	+
Phonological and orthographic measures																		
Phonological Awareness Composite	X	X	X	X	X	X	X	X	X	+	X	X	X	+	X	X	+	+
Phonological Fluency Composite	X	X	X	X	+	X	X	X	+	X	+	+	X	X	+	+	+	+
Orthography Composite	X	X	X	X	X	+	+	X	X	+	+	+	+	+	+	X	+	+
Neuroimaging - WORDS																		
[PDT and CDT]				X	X		X	X			X					X		X
[PDT, CDT and MDT]																	X	
[CDT]												X						
[PDT, CDT and VDT]	X	X	X			X			X	X			X	X	X			

Note: **X** denotes deviant performance (≤ - 1.65 SD below the mean of controls tested in this study); + denotes non-deviant performance; * denotes z-score (relative to the control group used in this study); The following subgroups of DPs have similar profiles on the behavioural composite and summary variables: Subgroup 1 (DP9, DP14, DP15 and DP17); Subgroup 2 (DP4 and DP8); Subgroup 3 (DP2 and DP16); Subgroup 4 (DP12 and DP13) and Subgroup 5 (DP1 and DP5); [PDT and CDT] denotes that the neuroimaging results are in agreement with the predictions of the PDT and CDT. [PDT, CDT and MDT] denotes that the neuroimaging results are consistent with all three main theories; [CDT] denotes that the neuroimaging results are in line with only the CDT; [PDT, CDT and VDT] denotes that the neuroimaging results are in line with predictions of the PDT, CDT and VDT (but not the visual MDT)].

Subgroup 5 (DP1 and DP5) was of special interest because although both DPs reported a history of difficulties with literacy, they did not show any deficits on the behavioural literacy measures. Despite being apparently well compensated on the behavioural measures, they both exhibited underactivation on the neural level. Their results suggest that although DPs can be compensated on the behavioural level, this does not mean that they are compensated on the neural level.

Summarising, DPs who have similar profiles on the behavioural measures can have similar profiles on the neural level, however in the subgroups examined above, a larger number of DPs with a similar behavioural profile exhibited dissimilar, rather than similar, profiles on the neural level.

It should be borne in mind that similar profiles on the neural level should be understood in the sense that they show underactivation consistent with a given theory, but do not necessary involve the same brain areas. For instance, the neural correlates of DP9 and DP14's (from Subgroup 1) word reading were consistent with the predictions of the PDT, CDT, and VDT. However, underactivation only in two frontal areas associated with the PDT overlapped in both DPs, but underactivation in four posterior and temporal areas did not overlap. Furthermore, whereas underactivation in three visual areas overlapped, it did not overlap in two other visual areas. Finally, underactivation in four cerebellar areas overlapped, but did not overlap in one cerebellar area.

5. Conclusion and Future Directions

Despite decades of research on dyslexia there is little consensus on the neural correlates of reading impairment in this developmental disorder. The main goal of this project was to shed more light on the neural correlates of reading deficit in adults with dyslexia, as hypothesised by the PDT, visual MDT and CDT, with special emphasis on individual differences among DPs. As reviewed in the Introduction, the majority of behavioural and neuroimaging studies, motivated by these theories, have three shortcomings. Firstly, they mostly tested one underlying cause of reading impairment in dyslexia. Secondly, they mostly relied on group comparisons. Thirdly, a significant number of these studies focused on detecting a deficit, hypothesised by a given theory of dyslexia, without empirically demonstrating the relationship of this deficit to reading impairment.

The research presented in this chapter addressed these problems. First, by contrasting the predictions of the neural correlates of reading impairment in dyslexia, postulated by each of the theories, in one sample of DPs. Second by using a multiple case study to investigate BOLD for each DP in comparison to the BOLD of CPs, thereby detecting differences which otherwise would have been obscured in the between-group comparison, due to heterogeneity among DPs. Third, by demonstrating a possible relationship between reading impairment and the neural correlates predicted by the main theories of dyslexia, using fMRI and a reading task.

The neuroimaging results for reading revealed that DPs exhibited complex and heterogeneous patterns of hypoactivation in the areas predicted by the three main theories of dyslexia. For instance, DP1 exhibited underactivation in eight areas predicted by the PDT (L Area 6 (BA6), L Area 44 (BA44), L middle temporal gyrus (BA21), L fusiform gyrus (BA19/37), L TE 3 (part of BA22), L IPC (PF) (BA40), L IPC (PFcm) (BA40) and L IPC (PGp) (BA39)), one area predicted by the visual MDT (R hOC5 (V5/MT)) and three areas predicted by the CDT (R Lobule VIIa Crus I (Hem), L Lobule VIIa Crus II (Hem) and R Lobule VIIa Crus II (Hem)). DP10 shows underactivation in one area predicted by the PDT (L IPC (PFm) (BA40)) and four areas predicted by the CDT (L Lobule VIIa Crus I (Hem), R Lobule VIIa Crus I (Hem), R Lobule VIIa Crus II (Hem) and R Lobule VI (Hem)). Finally, DP13 underactivated only areas predicted by the CDT (L Lobule VIIa Crus I (Hem), R Lobule VIIa Crus I (Hem) and R Lobule VIIa Crus II (Hem)).

Furthermore, the neuroimaging data showed a high degree of individual difference. Even if the neural correlates of reading deficit in two DPs are consistent with the PDT, the neural correlates in those DPs can be different. For instance, within the framework of the PDT, DP2 showed underactivation in L IPC (PF) (BA40), DP6 exhibited underactivation in the L Area 44 (BA44) and L IPC (PGp) (BA39), whereas DP7 underactivated L Area 6 (BA6) and L IPC (PFm) (BA40). This is also true about the neural correlates of reading which were in agreement with the CDT. For instance, DP1 showed underactivation in R Lobule VIIa Crus I (Hem), L Lobule VIIa Crus II (Hem) and R Lobule VIIa Crus II (Hem); DP14 underactivated L Lobule VIIa Crus I (Hem), R Lobule VIIa Crus I (Hem), R Lobule VIIa Crus II (Hem), R Lobule VI (Hem) and R Lobule VI (Vermis), whereas DP4 exhibited underactivation only in L Lobule VIIb (Hem). This could not have been uncovered with the traditional approach based on group comparison where only between-group differences (DPs versus CPs) are tested.

The results, showing considerable individual differences in patterns of underactivation within the reading network among DPs, are certainly surprising in the context of the between-group comparison studies, which have dominated neuroimaging research on dyslexia. However, they are perhaps less surprising if one reflects that reading is a human invention, relatively new in evolutionary history. Reading involves areas, which evolved for vision, language and associative learning. Reading acquisition is an exercise in brain plasticity, the goal of which is to create an efficient reading network which enables the unimpaired reader to get from visual precept to meaning in approximately 250 milliseconds (Pugh, 2006). Because of the number of areas involved, which have to be 'adapted' for reading in the ontogenetic development of an individual DP, perhaps it is not surprising that in different individuals with dyslexia, different components are impaired.

The neural correlates of reading deficit in dyslexia in all cases, except one, are consistent with the predictions of the PDT and CDT, in one case with the visual MDT (and PDT and CDT) and in ten cases with a hypothetical visual (not magnocellular) deficit theory (and the PDT and CDT). The underlying correlates of reading deficit in dyslexia are consistent with the predictions of only one theory of dyslexia in only one case – DP13 who exhibited results consistent only with the CDT. No DP exhibited reading deficit exclusively consistent with a phonological or magnocellular deficit. The underlying correlates of reading deficit in dyslexia in most cases are consistent with two or three theories and the CDT or PDT can account for all, but one case of the DPs.

The theories tested in this chapter (the PDT, visual MDT and CDT) have one important common feature – the assumption that one underlying deficit is necessary and sufficient to cause all symptoms of dyslexia: phonological, or visual magnocellular, or cerebellar, respectively. However, as discussed before, one of the shortcomings of dyslexia research is that it has mostly tested one underlying cause, guided by one theoretical framework. The results reported in this chapter clearly show that if one tests the same sample of DPs, contrasting the predictions of the main theories of dyslexia, the neural correlates of reading for most DPs are consistent with the predictions of more than one theory. In the sample studied here, the neuroimaging results for all, but DP13 are consistent with the PDT and CDT. Ten cases were also consistent with the VDT and one with the MDT. The protagonists of the PDT may argue here that the neural correlates of reading in these cases (except for DP13) are consistent with the core deficit in dyslexia, as hypothesised by the PDT, and that the underactivation in the cerebellum and/or visual areas in these cases just co-occurs with this developmental disorder. As emphasised above, in contrast to previous studies, this study, using fMRI, focused on the more direct relationship between reading deficit (the defining characteristic of dyslexia) and the predictions of the main theories on the neural level. It seems therefore that if some DPs exhibited underactivation in the areas hypothesised by the PDT and in the areas predicted by the CDT, during reading, it lends support to the claim that reading in these cases is consistent with the predictions of both theories and therefore both phonological areas and cerebellar areas contribute to the reading deficit in these DPs and the CDT effect is not just coocurring. Looking at these results from the perspective of the CDT, an additional interpretation is also possible, namely that the underactivation in phonological areas has been influenced by the cerebellum because the CDT predicts that a phonological deficit (in phonological awareness and in reading) can be caused by a cerebellar impairment. Hence, underactivation in the phonological areas in DPs (as compared to the CPs) can be consistent with the CDT (and the PDT). This interpretation, however, as pointed out earlier, is not consistent with the PDT.

Looking from a broader perspective at the issue of the neural correlates of reading deficit in dyslexia, a single deficit model has been prevalent for many years in the research on this and other developmental disorders. However, a single deficit model, although parsimonious and straightforward to test, has limitations. For instance, it cannot readily explain cases which exhibit a single deficit, but do not have a reading disorder. Such cases have been reported in longitudinal studies involving children 'at risk' of dyslexia (Pennington, 2011). Studies have also reported cases of CPs who, although exhibiting a phonological deficit, did not have a reading impairment (e.g., Reid et al., 2007). Furthermore, the single deficit model cannot account for comorbidities between dyslexia and some other developmental disorders which, as explained above, occur more frequently than would be expected by chance. Therefore a multiple deficit model has been formulated (Pennington, 2006).

According to the multiple-deficit model: 1) the etiology of complex behavioural disorders (such as developmental dyslexia) is multi-factorial and includes the interaction of multiple (genetic and environmental) protective and risk factors; 2) protective and risk factors modify the development of cognitive functions which are essential for the normal course of development, producing the behavioral symptoms that specify these disorders; 3) for a disorder to develop, no single etiological factor is sufficient, and it may be that several etiological factors are necessary; 4) because of shared cognitive and etiological risk factors, comorbidity (greater than chance co-occurrence) between complex behavioural disorders should be anticipated; 5) diagnosis for a complex behavioural disorder may be arbitrary because the liability distribution for such a disorder is usually quantitative and continuous (not categorical and discrete). Essentially the model is formulated within the same levels of explanation, as a single deficit model, such as the one proposed by Frith (1999), except that instead of the biological level there are two levels: the 'brain level' (neural systems) and the 'etiologic risk and protective factors level'. For more details on this model please see 'Future directions' section, below.

Some DPs in the study reported here exhibited hyperactivation. Overactivation in some DPs in the areas hypothesised to exhibit underactivation in DPs by the PDT suggests that a compensatory network is not limited to the frontal areas, as suggested by a number of studies involving exclusively group comparisons (e.g., Shaywitz et al., 1998), but involves areas distributed throughout the phonological reading network. Furthermore, in two cases, there were areas overactivated in the cerebellum, which points to the presence of a compensatory network within this brain structure.

Analysis of neuroimaging results for individual DPs in the context of reading scores revealed that lack of a clear deficit on a behavioural test (e.g., *TOWRE*) does not necessarily mean that the neural correlates of reading are intact. For instance, despite having a history of reading difficulties and a diagnosis of dyslexia, DP1 and DP5 exhibited no deficits on all the behavioural literacy measures, but their neural correlates of word reading, clearly showed underactivation. Furthermore, DPs who have a similar profile on behavioural literacy, phonological and orthographic measures can have similar profiles on the neural level, but not necessarily; in the subgroups examined in this chapter, a much larger number of DPs with similar behavioural profiles exhibited dissimilar profiles on the neural level. These findings further underscore heterogeneity among DPs.

5.1 Shortcomings

Historically, the main theoretical approaches to studying dyslexia (the PDT, the visual MDT and the CDT) were developed as separate and competing theories of dyslexia. Over the years different versions of these theories have been developed. For instance, a more recent version of the MDT (Stein, 2001) states that the cerebellum can be considered to be the most important part of the magnocellular timing system.

The focus of this chapter was on the well-established and most prominent versions of these theories, as described in the Introduction and this is both the strength and the weakness of the approach taken in this chapter. The strength of this approach lies in the fact that the predictions made on the basis of these versions are clear cut and differentiate the theories quite well. The weakness comes from the fact that the new theoretical developments within these theories may be omitted. However, it is felt that they are less well theoretically developed. For instance, it is not clear how the cerebellum can be considered to be the most important part of the magnocellular timing system because there are no magnocellular neurons in the cerebellum. It is becoming increasingly apparent that the neural correlates of reading impairment in dyslexia involve more than just one system, including the visual, the phonological and cerebellar processing systems, and in this new context, these theories can often be viewed as complementary, rather than competing.

A shortcoming which is unavoidable at present is the fact that not all areas of interest were labelled with the AT V.1.8. This is because probabilistic cytoarchitectonic maps have not yet been published for all brain areas. As a consequence two areas (L middle temporal gyrus and L fusiform gyrus) were labelled using perhaps the less reliable method (Tzourio-Mazoyer et al., 2002) which does not rely on probabilistic cytoarchitectonic maps.

Another shortcoming is related to the role of brain areas in a given process. For instance, many brain areas have been implicated in phonological processing, as reviewed in the Introduction, but it is not clear whether some of them are crucial for phonological processing, or they are just co-activated with other brain areas which are indispensable for phonological processing. Furthermore, the list of areas crucial for a given process is open-ended and as the research progresses, it may be that new areas will be discovered. Therefore the evaluation of a given theory may need to be updated in future research.

The study presented in this chapter is a cross-sectional study. Although such studies are valuable as they provide insight into a neural and/or cognitive system at a given time, one needs to bear in mind that if adults with developmental disorders are studied, there is a possibility that their neural system may have been significantly or partially altered due to compensatory mechanisms. The other possibility is that a given deficit is present during reading acquisition and influences this process, but is not detectable or is very difficult to detect in adulthood. Finally, it is possible that a given brain area was impaired and involved in reading acquisition but is not involved in adult reading. Therefore, longitudinal studies starting with infants with familial risk of dyslexia and control infants are indispensable in investigation of this developmental disorder (Goswami, 2003; Karmiloff-Smith, 1998; Ramus, 2004).

Although a detailed history was taken from participants regarding potential impairments (including developmental disorders), and measures for ADHD and DCD, no measures were recorded for other developmental disorders, which also tend to co-occur with dyslexia, such as, SLI (Specific Language Impairment) and SSD (Speech Sound Disorder). It has been reported that dyslexia is comorbid with SLI (Catts, Adlof, Hogan, and Weismer, 2005; Riccio and Hynd, 1993), approximately 30% of individuals with dyslexia also have SLI (Riccio and Hynd, 1993); more recent estimates are even higher (43-55%) (Newbury et al., 2011).

Extensive behavioural research has demonstrated that individuals who exhibited SSD in childhood are characterised by an increased risk of literacy difficulties (e.g., Aram, Ekelman, and Nation, 1984; Bishop and Adams, 1990; Catts, Fey, Tomblin, and Zhang, 2002; Hall and Tomblin, 1978; Scarborough and Dobrich, 1990; Snowling, Bishop, and Stothard, 2000). These studies also showed that approximately 30% of children with SSD develop literacy difficulties. Therefore it is possible that some sub-threshold symptoms associated with SLI and/or SSD were present in the DPs tested in this study. Future studies on dyslexia will need to include a larger number of measures of potential developmental disorders comorbid with dyslexia, including SLI and SSD.

As for many studies on dyslexia, the study reported here is based on a relatively small sample which consists of university students and therefore cannot be treated as a representative sample of the population with dyslexia. There is an urgent need in future research to rely on representative samples of DPs (Hulme and Snowling, 2009).

5.2 Future Directions

The neuroimaging findings reported in this chapter suggest that neuroimaging plays and will continue to play an important role in attempts to uncover the neural correlates of the reading impairment in dyslexia. One promising way forward in establishing the neuronal correlates of reading impairment in dyslexia, within the neuroimaging domain, would be to use various neuroimaging techniques. It is of crucial importance however, that they are used with the same sample of DPs and the emphasis of the research is on the individual differences among DPs. Multimodal neuroimaging could enable integration of measurements of high spatial resolution (e.g. fMRI) and temporal resolution (e.g., MEG), potentially providing better characterisation of deficits in dyslexia (Mathiak and Fallgatter, 2005).

Additionally, using other neuroimaging methods, such as structural MRI, MRS (Magnetic Resonance Spectroscopy) and DTI (Diffusion Tensor Imaging) with the same sample of DPs would allow for fuller characterisation of DPs' neural profiles. Although these neuroimaging methods may be interrelated, each method provides a window into a unique aspect of brain functionality. For instance, a recent MRS study (Pugh et al., 2014) is the first to test the role of multiple metabolites in developing readers. The authors reported an inverse relationship between both choline and glutamate and reading levels, such that higher concentrations of these metabolites were associated with lower scores. Given that heightened levels of choline are hypothesised to be associated with abnormal white matter organization (Gass and Richards, 2013), whereas heightened levels of glutamate can reflect hyperexcitability (Carrey, MacMaster, Sparkes, Khan, and Kusumakar, 2002), the results reported by Pugh et al. (2014) suggest potential links between abnormal white matter organization and reading deficit, and hyperexcitability and reading deficit in atypical brain development and reading acquisition.

Although the neuroimaging data provide a description of endophenotypes in dyslexia, they do not provide an explanation of what causes such endophenotypes. For instance, in this chapter the explanatory frameworks from the main theories of dyslexia were contrasted, however a deeper level of explanation at the genetic level was not addressed. Given the remarkable achievements of the Human Genome Project (Human Genome Project, 2011; Robbins and Stavroula, 2011) and the genetic studies of dyslexia, reported in the Introduction, genetics cannot be ignored in future studies on dyslexia, and will serve as an important branch of knowledge in future research on the neural underlying causes of reading impairment in this developmental disorder.

Indeed, the most recent studies which have combined neuroimaging methods with genetic data on variants of dyslexia risk genes (Cope et al., 2012; Darki, Peyrard-Janvid, Matsson, Kere, and Klingberg, 2012; Pinel et al., 2012; Scerri et al., 2012; Wilcke et al., 2012) have revealed that this new approach is fruitful. For instance, Cope et al. (2012) tested the association of fourteen variants in *DCDC2*, *KIAA0319*, and *TTRAP* with activation of sixteen brain regions of interest during an fMRI reading task. The strongest association occurred between complex tandem repeat BV677278 in *DCDC2* and activation of the L anterior inferior parietal lobe – an area for which previous neuroimaging studies have reported underactivation in DPs. Another fMRI study (Pinel et al., 2012) investigated the association of genetic polymorphisms with brain activation and functional asymmetry in frontal and temporal areas during a reading task. (Asymmetry maps were calculated by subtracting the activation of the R hemisphere from the corresponding activation in the L hemisphere). The authors reported three findings. First, single-nucleotide polymorphism (SNP) rs17243157 in the *KIAA0319/TTRAP/THEM2* locus was associated with asymmetry in the functional activation of the superior temporal sulcus. Second, SNPs rs6980093 and rs7799109 (in *FOXP2*) were associated with variations of activation in the L frontal cortex. Third, reading unimpaired participants who exhibited *KIAA0319/TTRAP/THEM2* variants showed a reduced L-hemispheric asymmetry of the superior temporal sulcus. Furthermore, a structural MRI study (Darki et al., 2012) reported that *DYX1C1*, *DCDC2* and *KIAA0319* contained SNPs that significantly correlated with white matter volume in the L temporo-parietal area and that white matter volume influenced reading ability in a sample of 76 young adults and children from the general population.

Finally, the focus is on DTI in the context of imaging the genetics in dyslexia. Although some interesting results have emerged from studies using DTI and behavioural measures in samples of non-impaired readers and DPs (Carter et al., 2009; Deutsch et al., 2005; Frye et al., 2008; Hoeft et al., 2011; Keller and Just, 2009; Klingberg et al., 2000; Niogi and McCandliss, 2006; Odegard, Farris, Ring, McColl, and Black, 2009; Richards et al., 2008; Rimrodt, Peterson, Denckla, Kaufmann, and Cutting, 2010; Steinbrink et al., 2008; Vandermosten et al., 2012), this technique could become particularly important when combined with genetic measures. This is because, as described in the Introduction, there is evidence that suggests that some dyslexia risk candidate genes are involved in impaired neuronal migration and neurite outgrowth.

The genes associated with neuronal migration (together with the environment and gene by environment interaction) shape structural connectivity of the brain which can be measured with DTI. One of the first studies (Scerri et al., 2012), which combined behavioural, genetic and DTI measures, reported that *MRPL19/C2ORF3* (locus on the chromosome 2p12, originally reported in connection with dyslexia) was associated with general cognitive ability in DPs and participants with SLI. Furthermore, associations between white matter structure measured using DTI and genotypes at the *MRPL19/C2ORF3* (in an independent sample) were found in the posterior corpus callosum and cingulum connecting significant parts of the temporal, parietal and occipital areas. The authors interpreted these findings as supporting the claim that the *MRPL19/C2ORF3* locus contains genetic variants which influence the white matter structure (in areas specified above), and this in turn influences the development of general cognitive abilities.

Although the field of imaging-genetics is relatively young and most findings need to be replicated, endophenotypes uncovered by neuroimaging hold a promise for building an important link between the behavioural and genetic characteristics of DPs (Carrion-Castillo, Franke, and Fisher, 2013). However, two shortcomings of these studies need to be mentioned here. First, these studies relied on dyslexia candidate genes and their variants discovered in neurobehavioral genetic studies. Although informative and interesting results emerged, they cannot test other genetic impacts on the overall reading deficits in dyslexia. Genome-wide association studies and sequencing studies are needed, so that new genes associated with risk of dyslexia can be discovered and their role tested in the neuroimaging studies, providing a fuller picture of phenotypes and endophenotypes of reading impairment in dyslexia (Eicher and Gruen, 2013). Second, as with the behavioural and neuroimaging studies reported in the Introduction of this chapter, the majority of studies which have combined neuroimaging methods with genetic data, have relied on group effects.

One of the challenges for future studies, is to focus on individual differences between DPs, and take into account many more different sources of variability which characterise DPs. For instance, the variability due to risk and protective factors in ontogenesis (e.g. the presence of an allele associated with dyslexia and good language skills, respectively), genetic variability, variability due to comorbidity with other developmental disorders, variability due to neuronal migration and axon growth, variability in structural connectivity and variability due to effective connectivity, to mention just a few. Given the considerable between-participant variability among DPs, future studies would need to rely on relatively large samples of DPs characterised by a considerable number of behavioural, neuroimaging and genetic measures in order to control for these variables. One of the ways forward would be to divide large samples into sub-samples of DPs with homogenous characteristics on independent behavioural, neuroimaging, genetic and environmental variables, so that they can be tested (separately from other sub-samples with different characteristics), for the underlying causes of the reading impairment. The variables which could not be controlled for, would need to be measured and entered into the analyses as covariates.

The complexity and multitude of factors involved in dyslexia has been addressed in a multiple-deficit model (Pennington, 2006) introduced earlier. The model accommodates the fact that there are multitudes of environmental and genetic risk factors and that they do not act independently (this is captured by bidirectional connections at each level). It may be that they are correlated with each other, or that they share effects of gene-by-environment interaction, or genes may interact with each other because they are part of the genetic system. As pointed out by Pennington (2006), the model does not specify the causal connections between the levels of analyses, including feedback loops from the behavioural level to the neural system level (or even to the etiology level). The strength and existence of causal connections will need to be determined via empirical investigation. Future research within this model, which focuses on individual differences between DPs and uses behavioural, genetic and neuroimaging measures, coupled with sophisticated statistical and modelling techniques, promises important insights into the underlying cause of the reading deficit in dyslexia and its comorbid disorders.

Appendix A - Tables for Introduction

Table 1. Results from the neuroimaging studies of phonological awareness, naming and short term memory in CPs and DPs

Study	Task	Imaging method	Results/Regions	Coordinates (x y z)	Z score
Phonological awareness, a sample from the unimpaired population					
				(Talairach)	
Paulesu et al. (1996)	Covert consonant rhyming: "Does *'p'* rhyme with *'t'* ?"	PET	L SMA (BA6)	-14 8 56	3.7
			L inferior frontal gyrus - BA44/45/46	-36 32 12	6
			(including Broca's area)	-46 12 12	6.5
			PMC (BA6)	-38 6 32	7.4
			L insula	-34 - 6 - 4	3.3
			L insula	-38 14 0	3.8
			L posterior superior temporal gyrus –	-46 - 26 4	6.1
			BA22 (Wernicke's area)	-44 - 32 12	3.9
			L caudate	-6 18 8	4.9

Table 1. (Continued)

Study	Task	Imaging method	Results/Regions	Coordinates (x y z)	Z score
			L caudate L cerebellum R insula R striatum R cerebellum	-22 22 12 -12 - 58 - 12 34 12 4 18 - 12 4 18 - 64 - 16	2.9 3.3 3.7 4.5 3.5
Booth, Wood, Lu, Houk, and Bitan (2007)	Word rhyming task with 3 words, e.g., 'hold – milk – cold', Ps were asked to indicate whether the final word rhymed with either of the previous two; which two items rhyme? Control task: line matching with three sets: '// - \\ - //'; Ps had to indicate whether the final set of lines was the same as either of the previous two.	fMRI	L inferior/middle frontal gyri (BA 46/45/9) L fusiform gyrus (BA 19/37) L superior/middle temporal gyri (BA 21/22) L putamen cerebellum (VI/Crus I)	-51 30 21 -45 - 60 - 21 -66 - 36 -3 -30 - 15 - 6 12 - 75 - 30 (not clear whether MNI or Talairach)	5.15 4.72 3.71 4.86 4.25
Xu et al. (2001)	Pseudoword rhyming relative to colour matching with letters	PET	L inferior temporal occipital junction (BA37) L Posterior-prefrontal cortex R Cerebellum L supramarginal gyrus (BA40)	-48 - 54 – 14 -44 4 28 32 - 68 20 -34 - 50 38 (not clear whether MNI or Talairach)	-

Study	Task	Imaging method	Results/Regions	Coordinates (x y z)	Z score
Covert object naming, the unimpaired population					
Lurito et al. (2000)	Covert naming of simple line drawings of common objects, relative to covert naming of abstract line drawings	fMRI	L inferior frontal gyrus (Broca's area) L posterior superior temporal gyrus (Wernicke's area) L posterior fusiform gyrus L middle temporal gyrus L middle temporal gyrus L premotor cortex L superior cerebellum R premotor cortex R superior cerebellum R supplementary motor area	-48 7 8 -50 - 39 17 -45 - 55 - 17 -55 - 43 -3 -53 - 28 - 4 -44 - 6 34 -32 - 50 - 20 51 - 7 32 35 - 50 - 21 2 - 6 49 (Talairach)	-
Moore and Price (1999)	Overt object naming, compared to saying 'yes' or 'okay yes' in response to nonsense shapes; Object naming compared to object viewing; Object naming compared to word naming;	PET	All comparisons elicited activation in: L anterior fusiform (BA20) L posterior fusiform (BA37)	-38 - 34 14 -40 - 50 - 12	3.3 3.4
Verbal short term memory, the unimpaired population					
Paulesu et al. (1996)	Ps were instructed to remember sequences of 6 consonants and 2 s later to make a judgement whether a	PET	SMA (BA6) L IFG (BA6/44) (Broca's area) L IFG (BA6/44) (Broca's area) PMC (BA6) L insula L STG (BA22) (Wernicke's area)	-2 2 56 -46 - 2 20 -42 10 16 -52 0 16 -36 - 8 36 -30 0 0	3.3 9.7 4.3 4.2 6.1 5.2

Table 1. (Continued)

Study	Task	Imaging method	Results/Regions	Coordinates (x y z)	Z score
	target consonant had been previously displayed.		L STG (BA22) (Wernicke's area) L supramarginal gyrus (BA40) L lingual gyrus (BA18) L cerebellum R IFG (BA6/44)	-46 - 38 16 -44 - 34 24 -14 - 68 -8 -12 - 68 -12 50 2 16	6.5 6.7 3.5 3.7 5.9
Phonological awareness, DPs vs CPs					
Paulesu et al. (1996)	Covert consonant rhyming: "Does *'p'* rhyme with *'t'* ?"	PET DPs<CPs	L prefrontal motor cortex (BA 6) L superior temporal gyrus (BA21/22) L insula R SMA (BA6) R striatum R striatum	-32 2 40 -44 - 22 4 -34 - 14 4 6 - 6 5 18 - 6 8 34 6 4 (Talairach)	2.7 1.9 3.3 1.7 2.4 2.5
Overt object naming, DPs vs CPs					
McCrory et al. (2005)	Overt object naming, compared to saying 'yes' or 'okay yes' in response to nonsense shapes; (also reading aloud, compared to saying 'yes' or 'okay yes' in response to false fonts).	PET DPs<CPs	L occipito-temporal region L occipito-temporal region	-48 - 54 – 16 -46 - 52 – 16 (unclear whether MNI or Talairach)	4.8 5.4
Short term memory, DPs vs CPs					

Study	Task	Imaging method	Results/Regions	Coordinates (x y z)	Z score
Paulesu et al. (1996)	Ps were instructed to remember sequences of 6 consonants and 2 s later to make a judgement whether a target consonant had been previously displayed.	DPs<CPs	L SMA (BA6) L inferior frontal gyrus (BA6/44) L PMC (BA6) L insula L SMG (BA40) L cerebellum R IFG (BA6/44) R insula	-8 0 56 -38 - 4 20 -40 - 6 32 -34 0 12 -46 - 44 24 -16 - 48 - 16 44 0 12 38 2 4 (Talairach)	2.2 4.2 2.2 3.9 2.8 2.4 3.3 3.8

Note: Ps = Participants; the macro-anatomical labels as specified in the cited papers.

Table 2. Results from the neuroimaging studies of V5/MT and other areas sensitive to magnocellular processing in CPs and DPs

Study	Task	Imaging method	Results/Regions	Coordinates (x, y, z)
V5/MT investigated in the unimpaired population				
Liederman et al. (2003)	Non-word reading with rTMS stimulation (experimental task) vs non-word reading with no rTMS stimulation (control task);	rTMS	Significantly more visual errors during the rTMS stimulation of V5/MT+ during nonword reading as compared to the control task	-
V5/MT investigated in DPs vs CPs				
Eden et al. (1996)	Ps viewed coherently moving, low-contrast random dots (Magno, experimental, stimulus) and a high-contrast, patterned stimulus (Parvo, control stimulus);	fMRI	All CPs exhibited bilateral motion sensitivity in volume search surrounding V5/MT; No DPs (except for one) exhibited activation in the same volume search;	L V5/MT: –52 ± 11, – 75 ± 8, 8 ± 5; R V5/MT: 50 ± 9, –70 ± 8, 5 ± 4;

Table 2. (Continued)

Study	Task	Imaging method	Results/Regions	Coordinates (x, y, z)
			All Ps exhibited similar responses to the control stimulus in the posterior occipital cortex (V1/V2) and extrastriate visual areas (inferior temporal/fusiform gyrus);	(Talairach)
Demb et al. (1997) and Demb et al. (1998)	Ps responded to moving visual grating stimuli presented at a low mean luminance, which stimulate magnocellular inputs to the cortex (Experimental condition); Ps responded (in the Control Condition) to contrast-reversing grating stimuli presented at a higher mean luminance;	fMRI	DPs significantly impaired in the following areas: V5/MT+ , V1,V2, V3, V3a, V4v DP not impaired on the control condition	-
Vanni et al. (1997)	'Magno task': the height contrast foveal stimulus, oblique black-white sinusoidal grating projected on the black background; It jumped abruptly to the right and then back once per 1.6 s; Ps were asked to fixate on a stationary dot presented in the centre of the display;	MEG	No sig. difference between the groups	LH: -33 ± 6, - 79 ± 9, 9 ± 7; RH: 34 ± 9, - 76 ± 11, 9 ± 10;

Table 3. Results from the neuroimaging studies which targeted the cerebellum in CPs and/or DPs

Study	Task	Imaging method	Results/Regions	Coordinates (x, y, z)	Z score
A sample from the unimpaired population					

Study	Task	Imaging method	Results/Regions	Coordinates (x, y, z)	Z score
Fulbright et al. (1999)	Rhyming judgement for pseudoword pairs	fMRI	R and L H lobule VI (simple lobule) R and L H lobule Crus I (superior semilunar lobule) R and L H Crus II and lobule VIIb (inferior semilunar lobule)	-	-
Fulbright et al. (1999)	Semantic category judgement for real words	fMRI	the same areas as for rhyming judgement (see above) R deep nuclear region the inferior vermis	-	-
Stoodley and Schmahmann (2009)	Language tasks (meta-analysis)	fMRI and PET	R H lobule VI R Crus I R Crus I/II R Vermal lobule VIIAt L H lobule VI	36 - 62 - 28 34 - 82 - 36 14 - 86 - 34 4 - 82 - 26 -42 - 58 - 24 (MNI)	12.18* 6.95* 9.91* 5.86* 6.36*
DPs vs CPs					
Nicolson et al. (1999)	Pre-learned sequence of finger movements *vs* rest	PET	CPs>DPs the R cerebellum	34^ - 40 34 (not clear whether MNI or Talairach coordinates)	3.75
Nicolson et al. (1999)	New sequence of finger movements *vs* rest	PET	CPs>DPs the R cerebellum	34^ - 46 34 (not clear whether MNI or Talairach coordinates)	4.38
Baillieux et al. (2009) (child DPs and child CPs)	A noun-verb association paradigm	fMRI	*Activation in CPs, absent in DPs:* R Anterior: H. lobule V (anterior quadrangular lobule) R Posterior: H. lobule VI (lobulus simplex) L Posterior: H. lobule VI (lobulus simplex) L Posterior: H. lobule VIIIA (biventral lobule)	25 - 49 – 22 29 - 64 – 19 -29 - 60 – 19 -24 - 60 - 40	-
Baillieux et al. (2009) (child DPs and child CPs)	A noun-verb association paradigm	fMRI	*Activation in DPs, absent in CPs:* R Anterior: V. lobule I and II/lingual	2 - 37 – 20	-
Baillieux et al. (2009) (child DPs and child CPs)	A noun-verb association paradigm	fMRI	R Posterior: V. lobule VIIAt,VIIAf/tuber, folium R Anterior: V lobule III/centralis R Posterior: Crus II (inferior semilunar lobule) L Anterior: V. lobule	5 - 75 – 28 7 - 49 – 25 30 - 63 – 38 - 13 - 54 – 17	

Table 3. (Continued)

Study	Task	Imaging method	Results/Regions	Coordinates (x, y, z)	Z score
			V/culmen L Posterior: H. lobule VI (lobulus simplex) L Posterior: Crus I)	 - 42 - 50 – 23 - 51 - 55 - 26	
Rae et al. (1998)	n/a	MRS (Magnetic Resonance Spectroscopy)	Cho/Na ratio (choline-containing compounds/N-acetylaspartate) sig. lower in DPs than in CPs	-	-
Laycock et al. (2008)	n/a.	MRS (Magnetic Resonance Spectroscopy)	DPs exhibited a higher ratio of Cho/Cr (creatine) in the L cerebellar hemisphere accompanied by a lower ratio of Na/Cho in the R cerebellar hemisphere	-	-
Laycock et al. (2008)	n/a	volumetric MRI	DPs had a larger volume of white matter in L and R cerebellar hemispheres;	-	-
Kronbichler et al. (2008) (teenage DPs and teenage CPs)	n/a	CPs>DPs Voxel Based Morphometry with T1 weighted MR images to investigate grey matter volume	R anterior cerebellum	27 - 54 - 33 46 - 46 - 33 (MNI)	4.88 4.22
Kronbichler et al. (2008)	n/a	As above	L anterior cerebellum	-34 - 41 - 31 -28 - 51 - 30 (MNI)	3.35 3.08
Brown et al. (2001) (adult men DPs and CPs)	n/a	Voxel Based Morphometry, comparing grey matter volume CPs>DPs	R and L semilunar lobules of cerebellum	18/-18 - 74 -38 -18 - 74 - 50	 4.30
Eckert et al. (2005) (child DPs and CPs)	n/a	Voxel Based Morphometry, comparing grey matter volume CPs>DPs	R cerebellar anterior lobe	-10 - 71 - 8 39 - 73 - 50 (MNI)	5.68 (t) 6.37 (t)
Eckert et al. (2005) child DPs and CPs	n/a	Voxel Based Morphometry, comparing white matter volume CPs>DPs	Cerebellar anterior lobe (analysis with white matter volume co-varied)	0 - 72 - 6 (MNI)	4.23 (t)

Study	Task	Imaging method	Results/Regions	Coordinates (x, y, z)	Z score
Pernet, Poline, Demonet, and Rousselet (2009) adult DPs and CPs	n/a	CPs' brains were used to build a 'typical' brain using bootstrapped confidence intervals. Each DP's grey matter was classified at each voxel as being outside or within the normal range.	R cerebellar declive (vermal lobule VI)	26 - 64 - 28 (MNI)	
Finch, Nicolson, and Fawcett (2002) 4 adults (except for one teenager) DPs' brains and 5 adult CPs' brains from the Orton Society brain bank.	n/a	Analysis of the size and density of cerebellar Purkinje cells; samples taken systematically from anterior, posterior and flocculonodular lobes;	*Cell size analysis:* Purkinje cells significantly larger in DPs than in CPs in the posterior cerebellar cortex; No significant differences in anterior and flocculonodular lobes; *Distributional analysis:* Significant differences in posterior and anterior lobes due to DPs having more large Purkinje cells and fewer small cells of this type; The dentate nucleus: no significant differences; Inferior olive: significant difference in distribution of cell sizes (due to fewer small cells and more large cells in DPs, when compared with CPs);	-	-

Note: R= right; L=left; H=hemispheric; * Activation Likelihood Estimate (ALE) values (10 to the power of -3, significant on a FDR ($p<0.001$); ^ x coordinate in the original paper is negative, indicating L cerebellum, but the label in Table 2 (original paper) states 'R cerebellum'; the first author confirmed that the R cerebellum was involved (personal communication – 29th of January 2010), therefore the negative x coordinate was changed here into positive x coordinate.

Appendix B - Tables (Local Maxima for Word Reading for Individual DPs)

Table 1. Local maxima for DP1

Brain area\Contrast	MNI			T	Z	voxels	probability	range from	range to
	x	y	z						
CPs>DP1									
underactivation supporting PDT									
Assigned to L Area 6	0	-6	68	6.56	3.88	582	90	80	100
Assigned to L Area 6	-2	2	58	5.7	3.62		80	0	80
Assigned to L Area 6	-8	4	50	5.53	3.56		60	40	70
Assigned to L Area 6	-36	-6	46	6.13	3.75	185	40	20	40
Assigned to L Area 6	-50	-10	46	5.84	3.67		50	40	80
L Area 4a							50	30	70
L Area 1							20	20	40
Assigned to L Area 6	-38	-6	64	2.74	2.28		40	10	40
Assigned to L Area 6	-12	-26	62	3.79	2.85	12	50	30	60
L Area 4a							40	30	50
L Area 6	-12	-14	60	3.42	2.67	8	60	50	80
Assigned to Area 6	0	-18	46	2.8	2.31	8	40	10	60
Area 4a							30	20	30
L Area 6	-30	-10	72	3.19	2.55		40	0	60
Assigned to L Area 44	-42	12	26	8.05	4.25	399	40	20	60
Assigned to L Area 44	-56	14	30	5.26	3.47		70	60	70
Assigned to L Area 44	-48	8	18	4.18	3.04		40	30	50
Assigned to L TE 3	-66	-34	20	5.22	3.45	528	50	0	60
L IPC (PF)							40	0	70
Assigned to L TE 3	-66	-24	0	3.23	2.57	11	40	10	80
Assigned to L IPC (PF)	-64	-42	24	6.22	3.78	528	80	60	80
L IPC (PFm)							40	0	40
Assigned to L IPC (PFcm)	-44	-36	26	6.38	3.83	113	50	0	70
Assigned to L IPC (PGp)	-26	-76	46	5.02	3.38	42	20	0	20
L fusiform gyrus	-44	-70	-18	3.84	2.88	46			
L middle temporal gyrus	-54	-16	-8	3.82	2.87	45			
underactivation supporting visual MDT									
Assigned to R hOC5 (V5)	50	-70	0	4.33	3.1	35	50	30	50
underactivation supporting CDT									
Assigned to R Lobule VIIa Crus I (Hem)	32	-82	-28	12.66	5.03	5420	100	98	100
Assigned to R Lobule VIIa Crus I (Hem)	28	-72	-38	11.19	4.83		88	50	88

Brain area\Contrast	MNI			T	Z	voxels	probability	range from	range to
	x	y	z						
CPs>DP1									
underactivation supporting PDT									
Assigned to R Lobule VIIa Crus II (Hem)	2	-84	-42	10.04	4.64		25	9	32
R Lobule VIIb (Hem)							14	0	14
Assigned to L Lobule VIIa Crus II (Hem)	-30	-70	-40	44.4	6.85	2249	83	19	88
L Lobule VIIa Crus I (Hem)							14	8	81
Assigned to L Lobule VIIa Crus II (Hem)	-22	-72	-38	41.98	6.78		76	9	76
Assigned to L Lobule VIIa Crus II (Hem)	-24	-82	-42	35.58	6.56		87	75	95
DP1>CPs									
nothing to report									

Note: Bold typeface denotes that a given activation peak was assigned to a given area (by the Anatomy Toolbox V.1.8) (AT) (Eickhoff et al., 2005); L denotes left; R denotes R; *'T'* and *'Z'* denote T and Z statistics (SPM5 output); *'voxels'* (SPM5 output) denote the number of voxels in a cluster; The AT uses probabilistic cytoarchitectonic maps (for more details see the section 'ROI analysis (mask)' above). To increase the reliability of the anatomical labelling, the probability at the corresponding voxel (see column *'probability'* in the table above) and the probability range for the surrounding voxels (see columns *'range from'* and *'range to'*) are calculated by the AT (Eickhoff et al., 2005). High probabilities are exhibited by a small number of voxels, in contrast small probabilities are exhibited by a larger number of voxels. This is the result of high variability in location and size of corresponding brain areas between different participants. As the volume increases, the probabilistic maps for different brain areas overlap at lower probabilities. Because of this overlap, some voxels of the reference space can be associated with more than one brain area. Therefore for some coordinates the probability and range are given for overlapping areas, not specified in the ROI mask. These are as follows: 1) L Hipp (CA) – L Cornu ammonis – one of the subdivisions of the hippocampus proper (Amunts et al., 2005); 2) Area 4a (an area in the primary motor cortex) (Geyer et al., 1996); 3) Area 3b and Area 1 (areas in the primary somatosensory cortex) (Geyer, Schleicher, and Zilles, 1999; Geyer, Schormann, Mohlberg, and Zilles, 2000); 4) L and R hOC3v (L and R Area V3v) and L and R hOC4v (L and R Area V4) – areas in the ventral visual cortex (Rottschy et al., 2007). For more details on these overlapping areas please see the publications cited above. Please see the section 'ROI analysis (mask)' for the correspondence between the labels assigned by the AT and Brodmann areas. As no probabilistic cytoarchitectonic maps are available in the AT for the entire *middle temporal gyrus* and *fusiform gyrus*, these were based on macroanatomically defined brain regions (Tzourio-Mazoyer et al., 2002). The results in Table 1 are reported at $p<0.05$ FDR.

Table 2. Local maxima for DP2

Brain area/Contrast	MNI			T	Z	voxels	probability	range from	range to
	x	y	z						
CPs>DP2									
underactivation supporting PDT									
Assigned to L IPC (PF)	-64	-42	22	5.53	3.56	8	80	0	80
underactivation supporting CDT									
Assigned to L Lobule VIIa Crus I (Hem)	-30	-70	-38	9.39	4.53	271	58	58	90
L Lobule VIIa Crus II (Hem)							42	1	42
Assigned to L Lobule VIIa Crus I (Hem)	-20	-76	-34	8.22	4.29	271	72	68	82
Assigned to L Lobule VIIa Crus I (Hem)	-40	-68	-38	6.3	3.81	271	53	53	92
Assigned to R Lobule VIIa Crus I (Hem)	26	-68	-40	8.04	4.25	104	49	12	51
R Lobule VIIa Crus II (Hem)							40	2	48
Assigned to R Lobule VIIa Crus II (Hem)	18	-74	-40	7.94	4.23	104	10	9	67
DP2>CPs									
nothing to report									

Note: The results in Table 2 (Appendix B) are reported at $p<0.001$ (uncorrected for multiple comparisons) to correspond to the results shown in Figure 1. Please note that activations for the L Lobule VIIa Crus I (Hem), R Lobule VIIa Crus I (Hem) and R Lobule VIIa Crus II (Hem) are significant at $p<0.05$ FDR. For other details please see the note under Table 1 (Appendix B).

Table 3. Local maxima for DP3

Brain area/Contrast	MNI			T	Z	voxels	probability	range from	range to
	x	y	z						
DP3>CPs									
underactivation supporting PDT									
Assigned to L Area 6	-6	0	62	5.05	3.39	181	80	60	80
Assigned to L Area 6	-2	-8	70	4.66	3.24	181	70	0	90
Assigned to L Area 44	-42	10	26	4.24	3.07	62	40	20	50
Assigned to L Area 44	-48	6	20	3.96	2.94	62	50	30	50
Assigned to L Area 44	-52	8	10	3.92	2.92	62	40	20	50
Assigned to L Area 45	-48	34	10	3.95	2.93	15	40	20	70
L middle temporal gyrus	-58	-62	2	3.88	2.9	26			
Assigned to L IPC (PF)	-64	-44	24	7.83	4.2	455	50	50	70
L IPC (PFm)							40	0	40

Brain area/Contrast	MNI			T	Z	voxels	probability	range from	range to
	x	y	z						
DP3>CPs									
underactivation supporting PDT									
Assigned to L IPC (PFm)	-60	-56	20	7.14	4.04	455	40	0	50
L IPC (PGa)							20	20	30
L IPC (PFm)	-52	-52	16	5.81	3.66	455	10	0	10
Assigned to L IPC (PGp)	-26	-80	46	4.94	3.35	21	20	20	20
L IPC (PGa)							20	20	20
underactivation supporting visual MDT									
Assigned to R Area 17	24	-98	-16	5.23	3.46	68	70	60	90
R Area 18							60	30	60
R hOC3v (V3v)							20	10	30
Assigned to R Area 17	18	-100	4	3.43	2.67	156	70	60	90
R Area 18							30	10	40
Assigned to L Area 18	-14	-96	18	5.53	3.56	43	50	30	60
Assigned to R Area 18	20	-66	14	4.82	3.3	110	40	20	50
R Area 17							30	10	30
Assigned to R Area 18	14	-66	20	3.58	2.75	110	40	10	40
Assigned to R Area 18	36	-92	-14	5.59	3.58	68	60	0	60
R hOC3v (V3v)							60	0	70
R hOC4v (V4)							20	0	30
R Area 18	8	-74	22	5.72	3.63	110	40	30	50
Assigned to R Area 18	22	-96	12	5.49	3.55	156	40	20	50
R Area 17							30	20	30
Assigned to R Area 18	20	-90	20	3.72	2.82	156	40	10	40
underactivation supporting CDT									
Assigned to L Lobule VIIa Crus I (Hem)	-30	-70	-38	17.1	5.5	1972	58	58	90
L Lobule VIIa Crus II (Hem)							42	1	42
Assigned to L Lobule VIIa Crus I (Hem)	-20	-76	-34	12.4	4.99	1972	72	68	82
Assigned to L Lobule VIIa Crus I (Hem)	-40	-68	-38	10.4	4.7	1972	53	53	92
Assigned to R Lobule VIIa Crus I (Hem)	26	-68	-40	8.58	4.37	2001	49	12	51
R Lobule VIIa Crus II (Hem)							40	2	48
Assigned to R Lobule VIIa Crus I (Hem)	32	-82	-26	7.78	4.19	2001	100	98	100
Assigned to R Lobule VIIa Crus II (Hem)	18	-74	-40	9.76	4.59	2001	10	9	67

Table 3. (Continued)

Brain area/Contrast	MNI			T	Z	voxels	probability	range from	range to
	x	y	z						
DP3>CPs									
nothing to report									

Note: The results in Table 3 (Appendix B) are reported at $p<0.05$ FDR. For other details please see the note under Table 1 (Appendix B).

Table 4a. Local maxima for DP4 (CPs>DP4)

Brain area/Contrast	MNI			T	Z	voxels	probability	range from	range to
	x	y	z						
CPs>DP4									
underactivation supporting PDT									
Assigned to L Area 6	-52	0	48	5.71	3.62	33	80	0	90
Assigned to L Area 6	-42	-10	46	5.13	3.42	33	40	20	60
L Area 4a							40	20	50
L Area 3b							20	10	20
Assigned to L Area 44	-48	6	18	7.42	4.11	32	40	20	50
L middle temporal gyrus	-54	-52	16	8.78	4.41	67			
L fusiform gyrus	-36	-44	-10	6.34	3.82	8			
Assigned to L TE 3	-66	-34	20	6.55	3.88	30	50	0	60
L IPC (PF)							40	0	70
Assigned to L IPC (PF)	-56	-32	36	7.72	4.18	80	60	30	80
L IPC (PFop)							30	20	30
L IPC (PFt)							30	20	40
L IPC (PFcm)							20	0	20
L IPC (PFm)	-62	-54	8	4.72	3.27	12	10	0	20
L IPC (PGa)							10	10	10
Assigned to L IPC (PGp)	-44	-72	22	5.88	3.68	10	60	40	60
L IPC (PGp)	-40	-62	10	7.68	4.17	27	10	0	10
L IPC (PGp)	-56	-68	14	5.27	3.47	14	20	20	30
underactivation supporting visual MDT									
Assigned to R Area 18	8	-74	22	8.04	4.25	58	40	30	50
Assigned to R Area 18	0	-74	16	5.51	3.56	58	60	10	60
Area 17							30	0	50
Assigned to R Area 18	24	-100	4	4.79	3.29	11	70	30	80
R Area 17							50	30	70
R hOC3v (V3v)							20	0	20
underactivation supporting CDT									
Assigned to L Lobule VIIb (Hem)	-14	-74	-50	6.19	3.77	11	74	26	80

Brain area/Contrast	MNI			T	Z	voxels	probability	range from	range to
	x	y	z						
DP4>CPs (see Table 4b)									

Note: The results in Table 4a (Appendix B) are reported at p<0.001 (uncorrected for multiple comparisons). For other details please see the note under Table 1 (Appendix B).

Table 4b. Local maxima for DP4 (DP4>CPs)

Brain area/Contrast	MNI			T	Z	voxel	probability	range from	range to
	x	y	Z						
DP4>CPs									
overactivation associated with PDT									
Assigned to L Area 6	-4	-6	74	5.62	3.59	7	60	0	80
Assigned to L Area 6	-4	16	50	4.92	3.34	6	50	20	50
Assigned to L Insula (Ig2)	-40	-18	-2	5.09	3.41	8	70	10	80
L IPC (PF)	-66	-36	2	5.29	3.48	14	10	0	10
DP4>CPs									
overactivation associated with PDT									
Assigned to L IPC (PFm)	-48	-48	48	5.4	3.52	73	50	0	50
L IPC (PF)							40	20	50
L hIP2							20	20	30
L hIP1							20	10	20
Assigned to L IPC (PGa)	-40	-60	52	5.73	3.63	73	50	40	60
L IPC (PFm)							40	30	40
L SPL (7A)							20	10	20
overactivation associated with visual MDT									
Assigned to L Area 17	-16	-66	8	6.58	3.89	59	50	40	70
L Area 18							30	10	40
Assigned to L Area 17	-20	-66	0	5.08	3.4	59	50	20	50
L hOC3v (V3v)							20	10	50
Assigned to L Area 17	-14	-84	0	5.33	3.5	11	30	10	70
L hOC3v (V3v)							20	10	50
Assigned to R Area 17	18	-84	12	11.3	4.84	232	70	40	80
Assigned to R Area 17	18	-56	2	4.94	3.35	26	90	70	90
R Area 18							30	10	50
Assigned to L Area 18	-12	-98	24	8.57	4.37	52	50	10	70
Assigned to L Area 18	-16	-98	14	6.25	3.79	52	50	50	70
Assigned to R Area 18	14	-78	-6	5.47	3.54	17	80	60	100
R hOC3v (V3v)							50	30	70
Assigned to R Area 18	14	-96	14	9.95	4.63	232	60	50	70
R Area 17							30	30	40

Table 4b. (Continued)

Brain area/Contrast	MNI			T	Z	voxel	probability	range from	range to
	x	y	Z						
Assigned to R Area 18	12	-86	20	4.81	3.3	232	40	10	70
overactivation associated with CDT									
Assigned to R Lobule VIIa Crus I (Hem)	38	-76	-26	5.85	3.67	9	100	84	100
Assigned to L Lobule VI (Hem)	-16	-64	-18	5.53	3.57	6	96	95	100

Note: The results in Table 4b (Appendix B) are reported at $p<0.05$, FDR. For other details please see the note under Table 1 (Appendix B).

Table 5. Local maxima for DP5

Brain area/Contrast	MNI			T	Z	voxels	probability	range from	range to
	x	y	z						
CPs>DP5									
underactivation supporting PDT									
Assigned to L Area 44	-42	12	26	5.51	3.56	8	40	20	60
L Area 45							10	0	20
L IPC (PFm)	-56	-50	18	4.64	3.24	8	20	0	20
L IPC (PGa)							10	0	20
CPs>DP5									
underactivation supporting CDT									
Assigned to L Lobule VIIa Crus I (Hem)	-20	-76	-34	9.68	4.58	321	72	68	82
Assigned to L Lobule VIIa Crus I (Hem)	-30	-70	-38	8.35	4.32	321	58	58	90
L Lobule VIIa Crus II (Hem)							42	1	42
Assigned to L Lobule VIIa Crus I (Hem)	-40	-66	-38	7.08	4.02	321	72	42	92
Assigned to R Lobule VIIa Crus II (Hem)	20	-76	-42	8.45	4.34	137	52	24	80
Assigned to R Lobule VIIa Crus I (Hem)	26	-70	-40	7.4	4.1	137	49	24	81
R Lobule VIIa Crus II (Hem)							40	2	67
Assigned to R Lobule VIIa Crus I (Hem)	46	-52	-36	5.37	3.51	13	100	91	100
Assigned to R Lobule VI (Hem)	36	-52	-32	4.94	3.35	13	59	44	90

Brain area/Contrast	MNI			T	Z	voxels	probability	range from	range to
	x	y	z						
DP5>CPs									
overactivation associated with the visual MDT									
Assigned to R Area 18	12	-80	-10	7.47	4.12	26	90	70	100
Area 17							20	10	40
hOC3v (V3v)							20	10	50
Assigned to L Area 17	-6	-102	0	5.2	3.45	11	90	90	100

Note: The results in Table 5 (Appendix B) are reported at p<0.001 (uncorrected for multiple comparisons) to correspond to the results shown in Figure 1. Please note that activations for the L Lobule VIIa Crus I (Hem), R Lobule VIIa Crus I (Hem), R Lobule VIIa Crus II (Hem) and R Lobule VI are significant at p<0.05 FDR. For other details please see the note under Table 1 (Appendix B).

Table 6. Local maxima for DP6

Brain area/Contrast	MNI			T	Z	voxels	probability	range from	range to
	x	y	z						
CPs>DP6									
underactivation supporting PDT									
Assigned to L Area 44	-42	10	26	7.46	4.12	17	40	20	50
Assigned to L IPC (PGp)	-28	-78	46	6	3.72	14	20	20	30
L IPC (PGa)							20	0	20
underactivation supporting CDT									
Assigned to L Lobule VIIa Crus I (Hem)	-30	-70	-38	10.8	4.77	252	58	58	90
L Lobule VIIa Crus II (Hem)							42	1	42
Assigned to L Lobule VIIa Crus I (Hem)	-20	-76	-34	8.61	4.37	252	72	68	82
L Lobule VIIa Crus II (Hem)							5	5	26
Assigned to L Lobule VIIa Crus I (Hem)	-40	-68	-38	8.04	4.25	252	53	53	92
Assigned to R Lobule VIIa Crus I (Hem)	26	-68	-40	7.02	4	93	49	12	51
R Lobule VIIa Crus II (Hem)							40	2	48
Assigned to R Lobule VIIa Crus I (Hem)	34	-70	-42	5.24	3.46	93	84	21	97
R Lobule VIIa Crus II (Hem)							15	0	74
Assigned to R Lobule VIIa Crus II (Hem)	18	-74	-40	9.81	4.6	93	10	9	67
DP6>CPs									
nothing to report									

Note: The results in Table 6 (Appendix B) are reported at p<0.05, FDR. For other details please see the note under Table 1 (Appendix B).

Table 7. Local maxima for DP7

Brain area/Contrast	MNI			T	Z	voxels	probability	range from	range to
	x	y	Z						
CPs>DP7									
underactivation supporting PDT									
Assigned to L Area 6	-6	2	62	5.18	3.44	12	80	50	80
L IPC (PFm)	-54	-54	18	5.52	3.56	8	10	0	10
underactivation supporting visual MDT									
Assigned to R Area 18	22	-96	12	4.57	3.2	7	40	20	50
R Area 17							30	20	30
underactivation supporting CDT									
Assigned to L Lobule VIIa Crus I (Hem)	-30	-70	-38	7	4	177	58	58	90
L Lobule VIIa Crus II (Hem)							42	1	42
Assigned to L Lobule VIIa Crus I (Hem)	-40	-68	-38	6.17	3.77	177	53	53	92
underactivation supporting CDT									
Assigned to R Lobule VIIa Crus I (Hem)	28	-72	-38	6.73	3.93	76	88	50	88
Assigned to L Lobule VIIa Crus II (Hem)	-18	-80	-36	7.55	4.14	177	89	26	94
L Lobule VIIa Crus I (Hem)							11	6	72
Assigned to R Lobule VIIa Crus II (Hem)	18	-74	-40	8.18	4.28	76	10	9	67
Assigned to R Lobule VI (Hem)	30	-54	-38	5.54	3.57	12	36	0	38
DP7>CPs									
nothing to report									

Note: The results in Table 7 (Appendix B) are reported at $p<0.001$ (uncorrected for multiple comparisons). For other details please see the note under Table 1 (Appendix B).

Table 8. Local maxima for DP8

Brain area/Contrast	MNI			T	Z	voxels	probability	range from	range to
	x	y	z						
CPs>DP8									
underactivation supporting PDT									
Assigned to L IPC (PGp)	-26	-80	48	5.51	3.56	6	20	0	20

Brain area/Contrast	MNI			T	Z	voxels	probability	range from	range to
	x	y	z						
CPs>DP8									
L IPC (PGa)							20	0	20
underactivation supporting visual MDT									
Assigned to R Area 18	36	-92	-14	5.68	3.61	15	60	0	60
R hOC3v (V3v)							60	0	70
R hOC4v (V4)							20	0	30
R Area 17							10	0	10
Assigned to R Area 17	26	-98	-14	4.67	3.25	15	60	50	80
R Area 18							40	40	80
underactivation supporting CDT									
Assigned to L Lobule VIIa Crus I (Hem)	-30	-70	-38	9.82	4.6	150	58	58	90
L Lobule VIIa Crus II (Hem)							42	1	42
Assigned to L Lobule VIIa Crus I (Hem)	-20	-76	-34	6.72	3.92	150	72	68	82
Assigned to L Lobule VIIa Crus I (Hem)	-40	-68	-38	6.42	3.84	150	53	53	92
Assigned to R Lobule VIIa Crus I (Hem)	26	-68	-40	8.8	4.41	192	49	12	51
underactivation supporting CDT									
R Lobule VIIa Crus II (Hem)							40	2	48
Assigned to R Lobule VIIa Crus I (Hem)	42	-78	-38	6.52	3.87	192	78	74	91
Assigned to R Lobule VIIa Crus I (Hem)	32	-82	-26	7.56	4.14	22	100	98	100
Assigned to R Lobule VIIa Crus I (Hem)	46	-52	-36	6.33	3.81	54	100	91	100
Assigned to R Lobule VIIa Crus II (Hem)	18	-74	-40	6.64	3.9	192	10	9	67
Assigned to R Lobule VI (Hem)	36	-52	-32	5.17	3.44	54	59	44	90
R Lobule VIIa Crus I (Hem)							41	9	56
Assigned to R Lobule VI (Hem)	28	-54	-36	5.23	3.46	10	77	11	86
DP8>CPs									
areas associated with PDT									
Assigned to L Insula (Id1)	-40	-14	-6	5.75	3.64	7	30	10	100
Insula (Ig2)							20	10	30

Table 8. (Continued)

Brain area/Contrast	MNI			T	Z	voxels	probability	range from	range to
	x	y	z						
DP8>CPs									
areas associated with visual MDT									
Assigned to L Area 18	-8	-86	-12	5.71	3.62	7	30	20	50
Area 17							20	20	30
hOC3v (V3v)							20	10	40
hOC4v (V4)							10	10	20
Assigned to L Area 18	-12	-102	10	5.09	3.41	15	70	60	90
Area 17							30	20	60

Note: The results in Table 8 (Appendix B) are reported at $p<0.001$ (uncorrected for multiple comparisons) to correspond to the results shown in Figure 1. Please note that activations for the L Lobule VIIa Crus I (Hem), R Lobule VIIa Crus I (Hem) and R Lobule VIIa Crus II (Hem) are significant at $p<0.05$ FDR. For other details please see the note under Table 1 (Appendix B).

Table 9. Local maxima for DP9

Brain area/Contrast	MNI			T	Z	voxels	probability	range from	range to
	x	y	z						
CPs>DP9									
underactivation supporting PDT									
Assigned to L Area 44	-42	10	26	7.12	4.03	95	40	20	50
Assigned to L Area 44	-48	6	18	4.99	3.37	95	40	20	50
Assigned to L Area 6	-6	2	62	5.11	3.41	57	80	50	80
Assigned to L IPC (PGp)	-26	-80	48	4.58	3.21	10	20	0	20
L IPC (PGa)							20	0	20
underactivation supporting visual MDT									
Assigned to L Area 17	-4	-80	10	4.7	3.26	62	80	60	90
L Area 18							40	10	50
Assigned to R Area 17	16	-102	4	5.24	3.46	91	80	70	90
R Area 18							30	20	50
Assigned to R Area 17	24	-98	-16	5.21	3.45	58	70	60	90
R Area 18							60	30	60
R hOC3v (V3v)							20	10	30
Assigned to R Area 17	20	-72	12	4.08	3	8	40	0	70
Assigned to L Area 18	-14	-96	18	4.92	3.34	26	50	30	60
Assigned to R Area 18	8	-74	22	6.23	3.78	81	40	30	50
Assigned to R Area 18	20	-96	12	4.3	3.09	91	30	20	60
R Area 17							30	30	40
Assigned to R Area 18	36	-92	-14	5.13	3.42	58	60	0	60
R hOC3v (V3v)							60	0	70

Brain area/Contrast	MNI			T	Z	voxels	probability	range from	range to
	x	y	z						
CPs>DP9									
R hOC4v (V4)							20	0	30
Assigned to R Area 18	28	-94	-10	4.49	3.17	58	70	40	100
R Area 17							40	20	50
R hOC3v (V3v)							40	20	60
Assigned to R Area 18	12	-78	-2	5.01	3.38	132	80	70	90
R Area 17							20	0	60
R hOC3v (V3v)							20	10	40
underactivation supporting CDT									
Assigned to L Lobule VIIa Crus I (Hem)	-30	-70	-38	12.4	5	1168	58	58	90
L Lobule VIIa Crus II (Hem)							42	1	42
Assigned to L Lobule VIIa Crus I (Hem)	-20	-76	-34	9.89	4.62	1168	72	68	82
Assigned to L Lobule VIIa Crus I (Hem)	-40	-68	-38	8.67	4.39	1168	53	53	92
Assigned to R Lobule VIIa Crus I (Hem)	26	-68	-40	7.33	4.08	640	49	12	51
R Lobule VIIa Crus II (Hem)							40	2	48
Assigned to R Lobule VIIa Crus I (Hem)	46	-54	-32	5.77	3.64	640	86	82	100
Assigned to R Lobule VIIa Crus I (Hem)	32	-82	-26	6.79	3.94	67	100	98	100
Assigned to R Lobule VIIa Crus II (Hem)	18	-74	-40	7.94	4.23	640	10	9	67
Assigned to R Lobule VI (Hem)	12	-66	-24	5.01	3.38	15	54	54	89
DP9>CPs									
nothing to report									

Note: The results in Table 9 (Appendix B) are reported at $p<0.05$, FDR. For other details please see the note under Table 1 (Appendix B).

Table 10. Local maxima for DP10

Brain area/Contrast	MNI			T	Z	voxel	probability	range from	range to
	x	y	z						
CPs>DP10									
underactivation supporting PDT									
L IPC (PFm)	-54	-54	18	6.01	3.72	10	10	0	10

Table 10. (Continued)

Brain area/Contrast	MNI			T	Z	voxel	probability	range from	range to
	x	y	z						
CPs>DP10									
underactivation supporting CDT									
Assigned to L Lobule VIIa Crus I (Hem)	-30	-70	-38	9.3	4.51	192	58	58	90
L Lobule VIIa Crus II (Hem)							42	1	42
Assigned to L Lobule VIIa Crus I (Hem)	-20	-76	-34	8.01	4.24	192	72	68	82
Assigned to L Lobule VIIa Crus I (Hem)	-40	-68	-38	7.24	4.06	192	53	53	92
Assigned to R Lobule VIIa Crus I (Hem)	26	-68	-40	7.12	4.03	110	49	12	51
R Lobule VIIa Crus II (Hem)							40	2	48
Assigned to R Lobule VIIa Crus I (Hem)	46	-52	-36	6.47	3.85	51	100	91	100
Assigned to R Lobule VIIa Crus II (Hem)	18	-74	-40	9.96	4.63	110	10	9	67
Assigned to R Lobule VI (Hem)	28	-54	-36	6.78	3.94	20	77	11	86
R Lobule VI (Hem)	36	-50	-32	6.02	3.72	51	75	59	96
R Lobule VIIa Crus I (Hem)							25	4	41
DP10>CPs									
nothing to report									

Note: The results in Table 10 (Appendix B) are reported at p<0.05, FDR. For other details please see the note under Table 1 (Appendix B).

Table 11. Local maxima for DP11

Brain area/Contrast	MNI			T	Z	voxels	probability	range from	range to
	x	y	z						
CPs>DP11									
underactivation supporting PDT									
Assigned to L Area 44	-42	10	26	7.04	4.01	49	40	20	50
Assigned to L Area 44	-48	6	20	4.35	3.11	49	50	30	50
Assigned to L Area 44	-52	8	10	5.02	3.38	16	40	20	50
L fusiform gyrus	-40	-42	-26	4.71	3.26	14			
underactivation supporting visual MDT									
Assigned to L Area 18	-14	-96	18	5.39	3.52	17	50	30	60
Assigned to R Area 18	20	-96	12	4.46	3.16	12	30	20	60
CPs>DP11									

Brain area/Contrast	MNI			T	Z	voxels	probability	range from	range to
	x	y	z						
underactivation supporting visual MDT									
R Area 17							30	30	40
underactivation supporting CDT									
Assigned to L Lobule VIIa Crus I (Hem)	-30	-70	-38	11.9	4.93	635	58	58	90
L Lobule VIIa Crus II (Hem)							42	1	42
Assigned to R Lobule VIIa Crus I (Hem)	26	-68	-40	13.8	5.17	543	49	12	51
R Lobule VIIa Crus II (Hem)							40	2	48
Assigned to R Lobule VIIa Crus I (Hem)	46	-54	-32	5.51	3.56	33	86	82	100
Assigned to R Lobule VIIa Crus I (Hem)	38	-56	-32	3.84	2.88	33	90	45	90
Assigned to R Lobule VIIa Crus I (Hem)	32	-82	-26	6.09	3.75	19	100	98	100
Assigned to L Lobule VIIa Crus II (Hem)	-20	-80	-38	11.2	4.83	635	91	79	98
Assigned to L Lobule VIIa Crus II (Hem)	-22	-72	-38	9.61	4.57	635	76	9	76
Assigned to R Lobule VIIa Crus II (Hem)	18	-74	-40	12.5	5.01	543	10	9	67
Asigned to R Lobule VI (Hem)	30	-56	-38	7.18	4.05	543	38	0	38
R Lobule VIIa Crus I (Hem)							14	0	57
DP11>CPs									
nothing to report									

Note: The results in Table 11 (Appendix B) are reported at p<0.05, FDR. For other details please see the note under Table 1 (Appendix B).

Table 12. Local maxima for DP12

Brain area/Contrast	MNI			T	Z	voxel	probability	range from	range to
	x	y	z						
CPs>DP12									
underactivation supporting PDT									
L fusiform gyrus	-40	-42	-24	5.79	3.65	16			
underactivation supporting CDT									
Assigned to L Lobule VIIa Crus I (Hem)	-30	-70	-38	12.6	5.02	330	58	58	90

Table 12. (Continued)

Brain area/Contrast	MNI			T	Z	voxel	probability	range from	range to
	x	y	z						
CPs>DP12									
L Lobule VIIa Crus II (Hem)							42	1	42
Assigned to L Lobule VIIa Crus I (Hem)	-40	-68	-38	8.82	4.42	330	53	53	92
Assigned to R Lobule VIIa Crus I (Hem)	26	-68	-40	7.07	4.02	98	49	12	51
R Lobule VIIa Crus II (Hem)							40	2	48
Assigned to R Lobule VIIa Crus I (Hem)	32	-82	-24	5.87	3.68	12	93	75	100
Assigned to R Lobule VIIa Crus I (Hem)	46	-54	-32	5.58	3.58	20	86	82	100
Assigned to L Lobule VIIa Crus II (Hem)	-22	-72	-38	8.37	4.32	330	76	9	76
Assigned to R Lobule VIIa Crus II (Hem)	18	-74	-40	8.38	4.32	98	10	9	67
Assigned to R Lobule VI (Hem)	36	-52	-32	4.54	3.19	20	59	44	90
R Lobule VIIa Crus I (Hem)							41	9	56
R Lobule VI (Hem)	28	-54	-36	5.78	3.64	9	77	11	86
DP12>CPs									
nothing to report									

Note: The results in Table 12 (Appendix B) are reported at $p<0.05$, FDR. For other details please see the note under Table 1 (Appendix B).

Table 13. Local maxima for DP13

Brain area/Contrast	MNI			T	Z	voxels	probability	range from	range to
	x	y	z						
CPs>DP13									
underactivation supporting CDT									
Assigned to L Lobule VIIa Crus I (Hem)	-20	-76	-34	8.34	4.32	201	72	68	82
Assigned to L Lobule VIIa Crus I (Hem)	-30	-70	-38	7.93	4.23	201	58	58	90
L Lobule VIIa Crus II (Hem)							42	1	42
Assigned to L Lobule VIIa Crus I (Hem)	-40	-68	-38	5.2	3.45	201	53	53	92
Assigned to R Lobule VIIa Crus I (Hem)	26	-68	-40	6.42	3.84	35	49	12	51
R Lobule VIIa Crus II (Hem)							40	2	48

Brain area/Contrast	MNI			T	Z	voxels	probability	range from	range to
	x	y	z						
CPs>DP13									
Assigned to R Lobule VIIa Crus II (Hem)	18	-74	-40	6.35	3.82	35	10	9	67
DP13>CPs									
overactivation associated with PDT									
Assigned to L Area 6	-2	16	50	5.37	3.51	8	50	30	50
L middle temporal gyrus	-50	-44	-4	6.15	3.76	7			
overactivation associated with CDT									
Assigned to L Area 17	-8	-102	2	4.63	3.23	6	80	60	100
Area 18							30	10	50

Note: The results in Table 13 (Appendix B) are reported at p<0.001 (uncorrected for multiple comparisons). For other details please see the note under Table 1 (Appendix B).

Table 14. Local maxima for DP14

Brain area/Contrast	MNI			T	Z	voxels	probability	range from	range to
	x	y	z						
CPs>DP14									
underactivation supporting PDT									
Assigned to L Area 6	-6	0	62	5.82	3.66	229	80	60	80
Assigned to L Area 6	-2	-8	70	4.33	3.1	229	70	0	90
Assigned to L Area 6	-10	-6	70	3.99	2.95	229	90	80	90
Assigned to L Area 44	-42	10	26	6.35	3.82	123	40	20	50
Assigned to L Area 44	-52	8	10	5.08	3.41	123	40	20	50
Assigned to L Area 44	-48	6	18	4.4	3.13	123	40	20	50
L middle temporal gyrus	-44	-52	18	4.26	3.08	100			
L middle temporal gyrus	-58	-62	2	4.05	2.98	68			
L middle temporal gyrus	-44	-50	-2	3.89	2.91	68			
L middle temporal gyrus	-50	-56	-4	3.7	2.81	68			
L middle temporal gyrus	-56	-8	-14	3.5	2.71	10			
L IPC (PF)	-66	-36	20	5.03	3.39	54	40	0	70
L TE 3							40	0	60
L IPC (PFm)	-54	-54	18	4.84	3.31	100	10	0	10
Assigned to L IPC (PGp)	-26	-80	48	6.29	3.8	18	20	0	20
L IPC (PGa)							20	0	20
L TE 3	-56	-12	-8	3.68	2.8	9	10	0	10
underactivation supporting visual MDT									
Assigned to L Area 18	-14	-96	18	4.69	3.26	21	50	30	60
Assigned to L Area 18	8	-74	22	5.14	3.43	19	40	30	50

Table 14. (Continued)

Brain area/Contrast	MNI			T	Z	voxels	probability	range from	range to
	x	y	z						
CPs>DP14									
Assigned to R Area 18	20	-96	12	5.62	3.59	128	30	20	60
R Area 17							30	30	40
Assigned to R Area 18	20	-90	20	3.4	2.66	128	40	10	40
Assigned to R Area 18	36	-92	-14	5.83	3.66	8	60	0	60
R hOC3v (V3v)							60	0	70
R hOC4v (V4)							20	0	30
underactivation supporting CDT									
Assigned to L Lobule VIIa Crus I (Hem)	-30	-70	-38	12.9	5.06	1394	58	58	90
L Lobule VIIa Crus II (Hem)							42	1	42
Assigned to L Lobule VIIa Crus I (Hem)	-20	-76	-34	10.6	4.74	1394	72	68	82
Assigned to L Lobule VIIa Crus I (Hem)	-40	-68	-38	8.7	4.39	1394	53	53	92
Assigned to R Lobule VIIa Crus I (Hem)	46	-54	-32	7.87	4.21	1230	86	82	100
Assigned to R Lobule VIIa Crus I (Hem)	32	-82	-26	7.85	4.21	1230	100	98	100
Assigned to R Lobule VIIa Crus II (Hem)	18	-74	-40	9.19	4.49	1230	10	9	67
Assigned to R Lobule VI (Hem)	12	-66	-24	4.37	3.12	52	54	54	89
Assigned to R Lobule VI (Vermis)	4	-64	-24	4.37	3.12	52	62	37	71
R Lobule V							18	1	28
DP14>CPs									
nothing to report									

Note: The results in Table 14 (Appendix B) are reported at p<0.05, FDR. For other details please see the note under Table 1 (Appendix B).

Table 15. Local maxima for DP15

Brain area/Contrast	MNI			T	Z	voxel	probability	range from	range to
	x	y	z						
DP15>CPs									
underactivation supporting PDT									
Assigned to L Area 6	-6	0	62	4.57	3.21	6	80	60	80
Assigned to L Area 44	-42	10	26	5.52	3.56	12	40	20	50

Brain area/Contrast	MNI			T	Z	voxel	probability	range from	range to
	x	y	z						
DP15>CPs									
Assigned to L Area 44	-48	6	18	5.03	3.39	11	40	20	50
L IPC (PGa)	-54	-56	18	5.13	3.42	19	20	0	30
L IPC (PGp)	-60	-60	22	4.73	3.27	19	30	0	30
L IPC (PGa)							30	0	30
underactivation supporting visual MDT									
Assigned to R Area 17	24	-96	-18	5.53	3.56	11	50	30	80
R Area 18							40	20	60
R hOC3v (V3v)							20	0	40
underactivation supporting CDT									
Assigned to L Lobule VIIa Crus I (Hem)	-30	-70	-38	11.5	4.88	349	58	58	90
L Lobule VIIa Crus II (Hem)							42	1	42
Assigned to L Lobule VIIa Crus I (Hem)	-40	-68	-38	8.17	4.28	349	53	53	92
Assigned to L Lobule VIIa Crus I (Hem)	-20	-76	-34	7.29	4.07	349	72	68	82
Assigned to R Lobule VIIa Crus I (Hem)	26	-68	-40	8.39	4.33	274	49	12	51
R Lobule VIIa Crus II (Hem)							40	2	48
Assigned to R Lobule VIIa Crus I (Hem)	42	-76	-38	5.49	3.55	274	86	72	86
Assigned to R Lobule VIIa Crus I (Hem)	46	-54	-32	5.91	3.69	87	86	82	100
Assigned to R Lobule VIIa Crus I (Hem)	38	-56	-32	4.91	3.34	87	90	45	90
Assigned to R Lobule VIIa Crus II (Hem)	18	-74	-40	9.44	4.53	274	10	9	67
Assigned to L Lobule VI (Hem)	-26	-52	-34	4.85	3.32	11	34	0	71
CPs>DP15									
nothing to report									

Note: The results in Table 15 (Appendix B) are reported at $p<0.05$, FDR. For other details please see the note under Table 1 (Appendix B).

Table 16. Local maxima for DP16

Brain area/Contrast	MNI			T	Z	voxel	probability	range from	range to
	x	y	z						
CPs>DP16									
underactivation supporting PDT									
Assigned to L Area 6	-6	0	62	4.8	3.3	6	80	60	80
Assigned to L Area 44	-42	12	26	5.67	3.61	8	40	20	60
L middle temporal gyrus	-58	-62	2	5.33	3.5	8			
L fusiform gyrus	-40	-42	-24	5.87	3.67	18			
Assigned to L IPC (PFm)	-60	-56	20	4.76	3.28	58	40	0	50
L IPC (PGa)							20	20	30
L IPC (PFm)	-52	-52	16	6.64	3.9	58	10	0	10
underactivation supporting visual MDT									
Assigned to R Area 18	20	-96	12	5.57	3.58	23	30	20	60
R Area 17							30	30	40
Assigned to R Area 18	8	-74	22	10.2	4.67	51	40	30	50
Assigned to R Area 18	20	-66	14	6.88	3.97	12	40	20	50
R Area 17							30	10	30
underactivation supporting CDT									
Assigned to L Lobule VIIa Crus I (Hem)	-30	-70	-38	10.7	4.75	288	58	58	90
L Lobule VIIa Crus II (Hem)							42	1	42
Assigned to L Lobule VIIa Crus I (Hem)	-20	-76	-34	7.47	4.12	288	72	68	82
Assigned to L Lobule VIIa Crus I (Hem)	-40	-68	-38	7.43	4.11	288	53	53	92
Assigned to R Lobule VIIa Crus I (Hem)	26	-68	-40	7.25	4.06	131	49	12	51
R Lobule VIIa Crus II (Hem)							40	2	48
Assigned to R Lobule VIIa Crus II (Hem)	18	-74	-40	10	4.64	131	10	9	67
Assigned to R Lobule VI (Hem)	28	-54	-36	5.02	3.38	8	77	11	86
DP16>CPs									
nothing to report									

Note: The results in Table 16 (Appendix B) are reported at $p<0.05$, FDR. For other details please see the note under Table 1 (Appendix B).

Table 17. Local maxima for DP17

Brain area/Contrast	MNI			T	Z	voxel	probability	range from	range to
	x	y	z						
CPs>DP17									
underactivation supporting PDT									
Assigned to L IPC (PGp)	-26	-80	48	6.76	3.94	9	20	0	20
L IPC (PGa)							20	0	20
underactivation supporting CDT									
Assigned to L Lobule VIIa Crus I (Hem)	-30	-70	-38	11.9	4.92	263	58	58	90
L Lobule VIIa Crus II (Hem)							42	1	42
Assigned to L Lobule VIIa Crus I (Hem)	-40	-68	-38	7.36	4.09	263	53	53	92
Assigned to R Lobule VIIa Crus I (Hem)	26	-68	-40	7.71	4.18	91	49	12	51
R Lobule VIIa Crus II (Hem)							40	2	48
Assigned to R Lobule VIIa Crus I (Hem)	32	-82	-26	6.43	3.84	12	100	98	100
Assigned to R Lobule VIIa Crus I (Hem)	42	-76	-38	5.95	3.7	28	86	72	86
Assigned to R Lobule VIIa Crus I (Hem)	46	-54	-32	5.56	3.57	18	86	82	100
Assigned to L Lobule VIIa Crus II (Hem)	-16	-82	-38	6.59	3.89	263	94	63	94
Assigned to R Lobule VIIa Crus II (Hem)	18	-74	-40	6.5	3.86	91	10	9	67
DP17>CPs									
overactivation associated with PDT									
L fusiform gyrus	-30	-52	-8	5.53	3.56	7			
Assigned to L Insula (Id1)	-40	-18	-6	6.27	3.8	15	100	50	100
L Insula (Ig2)							30	0	102
overactivation associated with CDT									
Assigned to L Lobule VIIb (Hem)	-18	-72	-48	4.82	3.31	8	84	68	84

Note: The results in Table 17 (Appendix B) are reported at p<0.001 (uncorrected for multiple comparisons) to correspond to the results shown in Figure 1. Please note that activations for the L Lobule VIIa Crus I (Hem), R Lobule VIIa Crus I (Hem) and L Lobule VIIa Crus II (Hem) are significant at p<0.05 FDR. For other details please see the note under Table 1 (Appendix B).

Table 18. Local maxima for DP18

Brain area/Contrast	MNI			T	Z	voxels	probability	range from	range to
	x	y	z						
CPs>DP18									
underactivation supporting PDT									
Assigned to L Area 6	-6	2	62	4.68	3.25	45	80	50	80
L Area 6	-10	-2	68	3.65	2.79	45	70	60	80
Assigned to L Area 44	-42	12	26	6.57	3.88	50	40	20	60
L Area 45							10	0	20
Assigned to L Area 44	-48	6	18	3.98	2.95	50	40	20	50
L Area 3b							10	0	10
L Area 45							10	0	10
L middle temporal gyrus	-44	-52	18	4.69	3.25	93			
L fusiform gyrus	-40	-42	-26	5.04	3.39	74			
L fusiform gyrus	-42	-50	-14	4.39	3.13	74			
L fusiform gyrus	-36	-26	-22	4.62	3.23	9			
L Hipp (CA)							10	10	20
L TE 3	-54	-16	-10	4.13	3.01	14	10	0	10
Assigned to L IPC (PF)	-64	-42	22	3.93	2.93	7	80	0	80
L IPC (PFm)	-54	-54	18	5.68	3.61	93	10	0	10
underactivation supporting visual MDT									
Assigned to L Area 18	-14	-96	18	5.03	3.39	24	50	30	60
L Area 17							10	10	20
Assigned to R Area 18	20	-96	12	6.41	3.84	145	30	20	60
R Area 17							30	30	40
R hOC3v (V3v)							10	0	10
Assigned to R Area 18	8	-74	22	5.08	3.4	35	40	30	50
R Area 17							10	0	20
Assigned to R Area 18	10	-70	-8	4.11	3.01	20	50	10	50
R hOC3v (V3v)							50	0	60
R Area 17							10	0	10
R hOC4v (V4)							10	10	10
underactivation supporting CDT									
Assigned to L Lobule VIIa Crus I (Hem)	-30	-70	-38	12.4	4.99	810	58	58	90
L Lobule VIIa Crus II (Hem)							42	1	42
Assigned to L Lobule VIIa Crus I (Hem)	-20	-76	-34	9.57	4.56	810	72	68	82
Assigned to L Lobule VIIa Crus I (Hem)	-40	-68	-38	8.76	4.4	810	53	53	92
Assigned to L Lobule VIIa Crus I (Hem)	46	-54	-32	6.91	3.98	845	86	82	100

Brain area/Contrast	MNI			T	Z	voxels	probability	range from	range to
	x	y	z						
CPs>DP18									
Assigned to R Lobule VIIa Crus I (Hem)	26	-68	-40	8.78	4.41	845	49	12	51
R Lobule VIIa Crus II (Hem)							40	2	48
Assigned to R Lobule VIIa Crus I (Hem)	32	-82	-26	7.9	4.22	96	100	98	100
Assigned to R Lobule VIIa Crus I (Hem)	20	-84	-28	3.57	2.75	96	94	94	95
Assigned to R Lobule VIIa Crus II (Hem)	18	-74	-40	9.55	4.56	845	10	9	67
Assigned to L Lobule VI (Hem)	-26	-52	-32	4.36	3.12	31	71	0	84
Assigned to L Lobule VI (Hem)	-34	-54	-28	3.68	2.8	31	85	76	95
L Lobule VIIa Crus I (Hem)							15	5	24
Assigned to L Lobule VI (Hem)	-14	-64	-18	4.1	3	7	95	94	95
DP18>CPs									
nothing to report									

Note: The results in Table 18 (Appendix B) are reported at $p<0.05$, FDR. For other details please see the note under Table 1 (Appendix B).

Appendix C - Tables (Local Maxima for Word Reading for DP8 and DP15; Analysis Searching for Possible DCD Effects)

Table 1. Local maxima for DP8 ('DCD analysis')

Brain area/Contrast	MNI			T	Z	voxels	probability	range from	range to
	x	y	z						
CPs>DP8									
parietal areas									
Assigned to L hIP1	-42	-56	48	5.73	3.73	16	50	40	50
L IPC (PFm)							40	0	60
L IPC (PGa)							30	0	40
L SPL (7A)							20	10	20
L hIP2							10	0	20

Tabe 1. (Continued)

Brain area/Contrast	MNI			T	Z	voxels	probability	range from	range to
	x	y	z						
CPs>DP8									
L hIP3							10	10	20
cerebellar areas									
Assigned to R Lobule V (Vermis)	6	-56	-16	7.37	4.23	178	45	45	82
Assigned to R Lobule VI (Hem)	14	-62	-18	4.01	3.03		93	92	95
Assigned to R Lobule VIIb (Hem)	30	-72	-50	5.37	3.6	8	44	2	72
R Lobule VIIa Crus II (Hem)							30	18	62
DP8>CPs									
parietal areas									
Assigned to L SPL (7A)	-18	-64	46	9.39	4.68	63	30	20	50
Assigned to L SPL (7A)	-12	-52	56	6.62	4.02	30	40	10	50
L SPL (5M)							30	10	30
L SPL (5L)							30	10	40
L SPL (7PC)							10	0	10
L Area 3b							10	0	20
cerebellar areas									
Assigned to R Lobule VIIIb (Hem)	16	-42	-48	10.5	4.88	138	40	3	40
R Lobule X (Hem)							27	4	78
R Lobule IX (Hem)							25	4	75
Assigned to R Lobule IX (Hem)	2	-46	-48	7.13	4.16	138	34	8	44
Assigned to R Lobule VIIIb (Hem)	22	-56	-50	4.8	3.38	138	59	45	60
R Lobule VIIIa (Hem)							24	5	26

Note: The results in Table 1 (Appendix C) are reported at $p<0.05$, FDR. For other details please see the note under Table 1 (Appendix B).

Table 2. Local maxima for DP15 ('DCD analysis')

Brain area/Contrast	MNI			T	Z	voxel	probability	range from	range to
	x	y	z						
CPs>DP15									
parietal areas									
Assigned to L SPL (7A)	-8	-60	62	5.09	3.5	94	60	30	70
L SPL (5M)							10	0	10
L SPL (7PC)							10	0	10

Brain area/Contrast	MNI			T	Z	voxel	probability	range from	range to
	x	y	z						
CPs>DP15									
L SPL (5L)							10	10	30
cerebellar areas									
Assigned to R Lobule V (Vermis)	6	-56	-20	5.95	3.81	558	14	14	76
Assigned to R Lobule V (Hem)	14	-46	-16	5.36	3.6	558	86	74	89
Assigned to R Lobule VI (Hem)	16	-70	-28	5.6	3.68	558	84	51	92
R Lobule VIIa Crus I (Hem)							10	6	49
Assigned to R Lobule VI (Hem)	36	-44	-38	4.07	3.05	15	77	26	86
R Lobule VIIa Crus I (Hem)							21	13	72
DP15>CPs									
nothing to report									

Note: The results in Table 2 (Appendix C) are reported at p<0.05, FDR. For other details please see the note under Table 1 (Appendix B).

Acknowledgments

The author is grateful to all participants with dyslexia and control participants who took part in this study. The the MRI scanning costs for this project were financed by the Lord Dowding Fund. Joel Talcott's help with this project is gratefully acknowledged. The author would like to express her gratitude to Liz Wilkinson (radiographer) for providing expert training on how to use an MRI scanner and helping with scanning participants. Thanks for the latter also extend to the Aston Neuroimaging Group. The author would like to thank Simon Eickhoff for making some additional probabilistic cytoarchitectonic maps available via the Anatomy Toolbox (AT) (these maps are now available in the AT V.1.8) and for advice in connection with the AT. Finally, the author gratefully acknowledges specialist advice on MRI and fMRI acquisition and analysis from members of the Aston Neuroimaging Group and the FIL Methods Group.

References

Albright, T. D. (1993). Cortical processing of visual motion. In: F. A. Miles and J. Wallman (Eds.), *Visual motion and its role in the stabilisation of gaze* (pp. 177-201): Elsevier.

Allen, G. and Courchesne, E. (2003). Differential effects of developmental cerebellar abnormality on cognitive and motor functions in the cerebellum: an fMRI study of autism. *Am. J. Psychiatry,* 160(2), 262-273.

American Psychiatric Association. (1994). *Diagnostic and statistical manual of mental disorders* (DSM-IV). Washington, DC: American Psychiatric Association.

Amunts, K., Kedo, O., Kindler, M., Pieperhoff, P., Mohlberg, H., Shah, N. J., Habel, U., Schneider, F., and Zilles, K. (2005). Cytoarchitectonic mapping of the human amygdala, hippocampal region and entorhinal cortex: intersubject variability and probability maps. *Anat. Embryol.* (Berl.), 210(5-6), 343-352.

Amunts, K., Malikovic, A., Mohlberg, H., Schormann, T., and Zilles, K. (2000). Brodmann's areas 17 and 18 brought into stereotaxic space-where and how variable? *Neuroimage,* 11 (1), 66-84.

Amunts, K., Schleicher, A., Burgel, U., Mohlberg, H., Uylings, H. B., and Zilles, K. (1999). Broca's region revisited: cytoarchitecture and intersubject variability. *J. Comp. Neurol.,* 412(2), 319-341.

Amunts, K., Weiss, P. H., Mohlberg, H., Pieperhoff, P., Eickhoff, S., Gurd, J. M., Marshall, J. C., Shah, N. J., Fink, G. R., and Zilles, K. (2004). Analysis of neural mechanisms underlying verbal fluency in cytoarchitectonically defined stereotaxic space--the roles of Brodmann areas 44 and 45. *Neuroimage,* 22(1), 42-56.

Amunts, K. and Zilles, K. (2001). Advances in cytoarchitectonic mapping of the human cerebral cortex. *Neuroimaging Clin. N. Am.,* 11(2), 151 – 169.

Anthoni, H., Zucchelli, M., Matsson, H., Muller-Myhsok, B., Fransson, I., Schumacher, J., Massinen, S., Onkamo, P., Warnke, A., Griesemann, H., Hoffmann, P., Nopola-Hemmi, J., Lyytinen, H., Schulte-Korne, G., Kere, J., Nothen, M. M., and Peyrard-Janvid, M. (2007). A locus on 2p12 containing the co-regulated MRPL19 and C2ORF3 genes is associated to dyslexia. *Hum. Mol. Genet.,* 16(6), 667-677.

Antonell, A., Del Campo, M., Magano, L. F., Kaufmann, L., de la Iglesia, J. M., Gallastegui, F., Flores, R., Schweigmann, U., Fauth, C., Kotzot, D., and Perez-Jurado, L. A. (2010). Partial 7q11.23 deletions further implicate GTF2I and GTF2IRD1 as the main genes responsible for the Williams-Beuren syndrome neurocognitive profile. *J. Med. Genet.,* 47 (5), 312-320.

APA. (1994). *Diagnostic and statistical manual of mental disorders (DSM-IV).* Washington, DC.

Aram, D. M., Ekelman, B. L. and Nation, J. E. (1984). Preschoolers with language disorders: 10 years later. *J. Speech Hear. Res.,* 27(2), 232-244.

Ashburner, J. and Friston, K. J. (1997). The role of registration and spatial normalization in detecting activations in functional imaging. *Clinical MRI/Developments in MR,* 7(1), 26–28.

Ashburner, J. and Friston, K. J. (2000). Voxel-based morphometry - the methods. *Neuroimage,* 11, 805-821.

August, G. J. and GarWnkel, B. D. (1990). Comorbidity of ADHD and reading disability among clinic-referred children. *Journal of Abnormal Child Psychology,* 1(1), 29–45.

Baillieux, H., Vandervliet, E. J., Manto, M., Parizel, P. M., De Deyn, P. P., and Marien, P. (2009). Developmental dyslexia and widespread activation across the cerebellar hemispheres. *Brain Lang.,* 108(2), 122-132.

Bates, T. C., Luciano, M., Castles, A., Coltheart, M., Wright, M. J., and Martin, N. G. (2007). Replication of reported linkages for dyslexia and spelling and suggestive evidence for novel regions on chromosomes 4 and 17. *Eur. J. Hum. Genet.,* 15(2), 194-203.

Benson, D. F., Sheremata, W. A., Bouchard, R., Segarra, J. M., Price, D., and Geschwind, N. (1973). Conduction aphasia: a clinicopathological study. *Arch. Neurol.,* 28, 339-346.

Bernard, J. A., Seidler, R. D., Hassevoort, K. M., Benson, B. L., Welsh, R. C., Wiggins, J. L., Jaeggi, S. M., Buschkuehl, M., Monk, C. S., Jonides, J., and Peltier, S. J. (2012). Resting state cortico-cerebellar functional connectivity networks: a comparison of anatomical and self-organizing map approaches. *Front Neuroanat.,* 6, 31.

Berquin, P. C., Giedd, J. N., Jacobsen, J. N., Hamburger, S. D., Krain, A. L., Rapoport, J. L., and Castellanos, F. X. (1998). Cerebellum in attention-deficit hyperactivity disorder A morphometric MRI study. *Neurology,* 50, 1087-1093.

Binder, J. R., Frost, J. A., Hammeke, T. A., Bellgowan, P. S., Rao, S. M., and Cox, R. W. (1999). Conceptual processing during the conscious resting state. A functional MRI study. *J. Cogn. Neurosci.,* 11(1), 80-95.

Bishop, D. V. (2001). Genetic influences on language impairment and literacy problems in children: same or different? *J. Child Psychol. Psychiatry,* 42(2), 189-198.

Bishop, D. V. and Adams, C. (1990). A prospective study of the relationship between specific language impairment, phonological disorders and reading retardation. *J. Child Psychol. Psychiatry,* 31(7), 1027-1050.

Bishop, D. V. M. (2002). Cerebellar abnormalities in developmental dyslexia: Cause, correlate or consequence? *Cortex,* 38, 491-498.

Black, J. E., Isaacs, K. R., Anderson, B. J., Alcantara, A. A., and Greenough, W. T. (1990). Learning causes synaptogenesis, whereas motor activity causes angiogenesis, in cerebellar cortex of adult rats. *Proceedings of the National Academy of Sciences, US,* 87, 5568-5572.

Booth, J. R., Wood, L., Lu, D., Houk, J. C., and Bitan, T. (2007). The role of the basal ganglia and cerebellum in language processing. *Brain Res.,* 1133(1), 136-144.

Braddick, O., Atkinson, J. and Wattam-Bell, J. (2003). Normal and anomalous development of visual motion processing: motion coherence and 'dorsal-stream vulnerability'. *Neuropsychologia,* 41(13), 1769-1784.

Bradley, L. and Bryant, P. E. (1983). Categorising sounds and learning to read - a causal connection. *Nature,* 301(5899), 419-421.

Brady, S., Shankweiler, D. P. and Mann, V. (1983). Speech perception and memory coding in relation to reading ability. *Journal of Experimental Child Psychology,* 35, 345-367.

Brett, M. (1999). *The MNI Brain and The Talairach Atlas*. Cambridge Imagers: http://www.mrc-cbu.cam.ac.uk/Imaging/mnispace.html.

Brett, M., Anton, J. L., Valabregue, R., and Poline, J. B. (2002). Region of interest analysis using an SPM toolbox, *The 8th International Conference on Functional Mapping of the Human Brain*. Sendai, Japan: Available on CD-ROM in NeuroImage, Vol. 16, No 2.

British Dyslexia Association. (2007). BDA definition of dyslexia. Accessed on line http://www.bdadyslexia.org.uk/about-dyslexia/further-information/dyslexia-research-information-.html on 12/06/2012.

Brockway, J. P. (2011). *Intraoperative basal temporal language maps.* Unpublished manuscript, Charlotte, NC.

Brodal, A. (1981). The cerebellum. In: A. Brodal (Ed.), *Neurological anatomy in relation to clinical medicine* (pp. 294-393). Oxford: Oxford University Press.

Brookes, R. L., Nicolson, R. I. and Fawcett, A. J. (2007). Prisms throw light on developmental disorders. *Neuropsychologia,* 45(8), 1921-1930.

Brown, W. E., Eliez, S., Menon, V., Rumsey, J. M., White, C. D., and Reiss, A. L. (2001). Preliminary evidence of widespread morphological variations of the brain in dyslexia. *Neurology,* 56(6), 781-783.

Bruck, M. (1990). Word-recognition skills of adults with childhood diagnosis of dyslexia. *Developmental Psychology,* 26(3), 439-454.

Brunswick, N. (2011). *Living with dyslexia.* New York: Rosen.

Brunswick, N., McCrory, E., Price, C. J., Frith, C. D., and Frith, U. (1999). Explicit and implicit processing of words and pseudowords by adult developmental dyslexics: A search for Wernicke's Wortschatz? *Brain,* 122 (Pt 10), 1901-1917.

Burbridge, T. J., Wang, Y., Volz, A. J., Peschansky, V. J., Lisann, L., Galaburda, A. M., Lo Turco, J. J., and Rosen, G. D. (2008). Postnatal analysis of the effect of embryonic knockdown and overexpression of candidate dyslexia susceptibility gene homolog Dcdc2 in the rat. *Neuroscience,* 152(3), 723-733.

Cabeza, R., Anderson, N. D., Locantore, J. K., and McIntosh, A. R. (2002). Aging gracefully: compensatory brain activity in high-performing older adults. *Neuroimage,* 17(3), 1394-1402.

Carrey, N., MacMaster, F. P., Sparkes, S. J., Khan, S. C., and Kusumakar, V. (2002). Glutamatergic changes with treatment in attention deficit hyperactivity disorder: a preliminary case series. *J. Child Adolesc. Psychopharmacol.,* 12(4), 331-336.

Carrion-Castillo, A., Franke, B. and Fisher, S. E. (2013). Molecular genetics of dyslexia: an overview. *Dyslexia,* 19(4), 214-240.

Carroll, J. M., Maughan, B., Goodman, R., and Meltzer, H. (2005). Literacy difficulties and psychiatric disorders: evidence for comorbidity. *Journal of Child Psychology and Psychiatry,* 46(5), 524–532.

Carter, J. C., Lanham, D. C., Cutting, L. E., Clements-Stephens, A. M., Chen, X., Hadzipasic, M., Kim, J., Denckla, M. B., and Kaufmann, W. E. (2009). A dual DTI approach to analyzing white matter in children with dyslexia. *Psychiatry Res.,* 172(3), 215-219.

Caspers, S., Eickhoff, S. B., Geyer, S., Scheperjans, F., Mohlberg, H., Zilles, K., and Amunts, K. (2008). The human inferior parietal lobule in stereotaxic space. *Brain Struct. Funct.,* 212(6), 481-495.

Caspers, S., Geyer, S., Schleicher, A., Mohlberg, H., Amunts, K., and Zilles, K. (2006). The human inferior parietal cortex: cytoarchitectonic parcellation and interindividual variability. *Neuroimage,* 33(2), 430-448.

Castles, A. and Coltheart, M. (1993). Varieties of developmental dyslexia. *Cognition,* 47 149-180.

Catts, H. W., Adlof, S. M., Hogan, T. P., and Weismer, S. E. (2005). Are specific language impairment and dyslexia distinct disorders? *Journal of Speech, Language, and Hearing Research,* 48, 1378-1396.

Catts, H. W., Fey, M. E., Tomblin, J. B., and Zhang, X. (2002). A longitudinal investigation of reading outcomes in children with language impairments. *J. Speech Lang. Hear. Res.,* 45(6), 1142-1157.

Choi, H. J., Zilles, K., Mohlberg, H., Schleicher, A., Fink, G. R., Armstrong, E., and Amunts, K. (2006). Cytoarchitectonic identification and probabilistic mapping of two distinct areas within the anterior ventral bank of the human intraparietal sulcus. *J. Comp. Neurol.,* 495(1), 53-69.

Cohen, L. and Dehaene, S. (2004). Specialization within the ventral stream: the case for the visual word form area. *Neuroimage,* 22(1), 466-476.

Cohen, L., Dehaene, S., Naccache, L., Lehericy, S., Dehaene-Lambertz, G., Henaff, M. A., and Michel, F. (2000). The visual word form area: spatial and temporal characterization of an initial stage of reading in normal subjects and posterior split-brain patients. *Brain,* 123 (Pt 2), 291-307.

Cohen, L., Lehericy, S., Chochon, F., Lemer, C., Rivaud, S., and Dehaene, S. (2002). Language-specific tuning of visual cortex? Functional properties of the Visual Word Form Area. *Brain,* 125(Pt 5), 1054-1069.

Cohen, L., Martinaud, O., Lemer, C., Lehericy, S., Samson, Y., Obadia, M., Slachevsky, A., and Dehaene, S. (2003). Visual word recognition in the left and right hemispheres: anatomical and functional correlates of peripheral alexias. *Cereb. Cortex,* 13(12), 1313-1333.

Coltheart, M. (1981). The MRC psycholinguistic database. *Quarterly Journal of Experimental Psychology,* 33A, 497-505.

Conners, C. K., Erhardt, D. and Sparrow, E. P. (1999). *Conners' Adult ADHD Rating Scales (CAARS).* New York: MHS.

Cope, N., Eicher, J. D., Meng, H., Gibson, C. J., Hager, K., Lacadie, C., Fulbright, R. K., Constable, R. T., Page, G. P., and Gruen, J. R. (2012). Variants in the DYX2 locus are associated with altered brain activation in reading-related brain regions in subjects with reading disability. *Neuroimage,* 63(1), 148-156.

Cope, N., Harold, D., Hill, G., Moskvina, V., Stevenson, J., Holmans, P., Owen, M. J., O'Donovan, M. C., and Williams, J. (2005). Strong evidence that KIAA0319 on chromosome 6p is a susceptibility gene for developmental dyslexia. *American Journal of Human Genetics,* 76(4), 581–591.

Cornelissen, P., Richardson, A., Mason, A., Fowler, S., and Stein, J. (1995). Contrast sensitivity and coherent motion detection measured at photopic luminance levels in dyslexics and controls. *Vision Res.,* 35(10), 1483-1494.

Couto, J. M., Gomez, L., Wigg, K., Cate-Carter, T., Archibald, J., Anderson, B., Tannock, R., Kerr, E. N., Lovett, M. W., Humphries, T., and Barr, C. L. (2008). The KIAA0319-like (KIAA0319L) gene on chromosome 1p34 as a candidate for reading disabilities. *J. Neurogenet.,* 22(4), 295-313.

Couto, J. M., Gomez, L., Wigg, K., Ickowicz, A., Pathare, T., Malone, M., Kennedy, J. L., Schachar, R., and Barr, C. L. (2009). Association of attention-deficit/hyperactivity disorder with a candidate region for reading disabilities on chromosome 6p. *Biol. Psychiatry,* 66(4), 368-375.

Crossman, A. R. and Neary, D. (2005). *Neuroanatomy.* London: Churchil Livingstone Elsevier.

Damasio, H. and Damasio, A. R. (1980). The anatomical basis of conduction aphasia. *Brain,* 103, 337-350.

Darki, F., Peyrard-Janvid, M., Matsson, H., Kere, J., and Klingberg, T. (2012). Three dyslexia susceptibility genes, DYX1C1, DCDC2, and KIAA0319, affect temporo-parietal white matter structure. *Biol. Psychiatry,* 72(8), 671-676.

Daum, I., Schugens, M. M., Ackermann, H., Lutzenberger, W., Dichgans, J., and Birbaumer, N. (1993). Classical conditioning after cerebellar lesions in humans. *Behav. Neurosci.,* 107, 748–756.

De Kovel, C. G., Hol, F. A., Heister, J. G., Willemen, J. J., Sandkuijl, L. A., Franke, B., and Padberg, G. W. (2004). Genomewide scan identifies susceptibility locus for dyslexia on Xq27 in an extended Dutch family. *J. Med. Genet.,* 41(9), 652-657.

Dechent, P. and Frahm, J. (2003). Characterization of the human visual V6 complex by functional magnetic resonance imaging. *Eur. J. Neurosci.* 17(10), 2201-2211.

Deffenbacher, K. E., Kenyon, J. B., Hoover, D. M., Olson, R. K., Pennington, B. F., DeFries, J. C., and Smith, S. D. (2004). Refinement of the 6p21.3 quantitative trait locus influencing dyslexia: linkage and association analyses. *Hum. Genet.,* 115(2), 128-138.

DeFries, J. C. and Alarcon, M. (1996). Genetics of specific reading disability. *Mental Retard. Dev. Disabilities Res. Rev.,* 2, 39-47.

DeFries, J. C. and Fulker, D. W. (1985). Multiple regression analysis of twin data. *Behav. Genet.,* 15, 467-473.

DeFries, J. C., Fulker, D. W. and LaBuda, M. C. (1987). Evidence for a genetic aetiology in reading disability of twins. *Nature,* 329(6139), 537-539.

Demb, J. B., Boynton, G. M. and Heeger, D. J. (1997). Brain activity in visual cortex predicts individual differences in reading performance. *Proc. Natl. Acad. Sci. US,* 94, 13363–13366.

Demb, J. B., Boynton, G. M. and Heeger, D. J. (1998). Functional magnetic resonance imaging of early visual pathways in dyslexia. *J. Neurosci.,* 18(17), 6939-6951.

Demonet, J. F., Taylor, M. J. and Chaix, Y. (2004). Developmental dyslexia. *Lancet,* 363 (9419), 1451-1460.

Denckla, M. B. (1985). Motor coordination in dyslexic children: Theoretical and clinical implications. In: F. H. Duffy and N. Geschwind (Eds.), *Dyslexia: A neuroscientific approach to clinical evaluation*. Boston: Little, Brown.

Denckla, M. B. and Rudel, R. G. (1976). Rapid "automatized" naming (R.A.N): dyslexia differentiated from other learning disabilities. *Neuropsychologia,* 14(4), 471-479.

Deutsch, G. K., Dougherty, R. F., Bammer, R., Siok, W. T., Gabrieli, J. D. E., and Wandell, B. (2005). Children's reading performance is correlated with while matter structure measured by diffusion tensor imaging. *Cortex,* 41, 354-363.

Devlin, J. T., Jamison, H. L., Gonnerman, L. M., and Matthews, P. M. (2006). The role of the posterior fusiform gyrus in reading. *J. Cogn. Neurosci.,* 18(6), 911-922.

Diedrichsen, J., Balsters, J. H., Flavell, J., Cussans, E., and Ramnani, N. (2009). A probabilistic MR atlas of the human cerebellum. *Neuroimage,* 46(1), 39-46.

Dietz, N. A., Jones, K. M., Gareau, L., Zeffiro, T. A., and Eden, G. F. (2005). Phonological decoding involves left posterior fusiform gyrus. *Hum. Brain Mapp.,* 26(2), 81-93.

Doyle, A. E., Ferreira, M. A., Sklar, P. B., Lasky-Su, J., Petty, C., Fusillo, S. J., Seidman, L. J., Willcutt, E. G., Smoller, J. W., Purcell, S., Biederman, J., and Faraone, S. V. (2008). Multivariate genomewide linkage scan of neurocognitive traits and ADHD symptoms: suggestive linkage to 3q13. *Am. J. Med. Genet. B Neuropsychiatr. Genet.,* 147B(8), 1399-1411.

Dykman, R. A. and Ackerman, P. T. (1991). Attention deficit disorder and specific reading disability: Separate but often overlapping disorders. *Journal of Learning Disabilities,* 24, 96-103.

Dyspraxia Foundation. (2012). Information accessed online: http://www.dyspraxiafoundation.org.uk/services/ad_symptoms.php, on the 15th of November 2012.

Eckert, M. A., Leonard, C. M., Richards, T. L., Aylward, E. H., Thomson, J., and Berninger, V. W. (2003). Anatomical correlates of dyslexia: frontal and cerebellar findings. *Brain,* 126(Pt 2), 482-494.

Eckert, M. A., Leonard, C. M., Wilke, M., Eckert, M., Richards, T., Richards, A., and Berninger, V. (2005). Anatomical signatures of dyslexia in children: unique information from manual and voxel based morphometry brain measures. *Cortex,* 41(3), 304-315.

Eden, G. F., Jones, K. M., Cappell, K., Gareau, L., Wood, F. B., Zeffiro, T. A., Dietz, N. A., Agnew, J. A., and Flowers, D. L. (2004). Neural changes following remediation in adult developmental dyslexia. *Neuron,* 44(3), 411-422.

Eden, G. F., VanMeter, J. W., Rumsey, J. M., Maisog, J. M., Woods, R. P., and Zeffiro, T. A. (1996). Abnormal processing of visual motion in dyslexia revealed by functional brain imaging. *Nature,* 382(6586), 66-69.

Eicher, J. D. and Gruen, J. R. (2013). Imaging-genetics in dyslexia: connecting risk genetic variants to brain neuroimaging and ultimately to reading impairments. *Mol. Genet. Metab.,* 110(3), 201-212.

Eickhoff, S. B., Stephan, K. E., Mohlberg, H., Grefkes, C., Fink, G. R., Amunts, K., and Zilles, K. (2005). A new SPM toolbox for combining probabilistic cytoarchitectonic maps and functional imaging data. *Neuroimage,* 25(4), 1325-1335.

Fawcett, A. J. and Nicholson, R. I. (1995). Persistent deficits in motor skill of children with dyslexia. *Journal of Motor Behaviour* 27, 235-240.

Fawcett, A. J. and Nicolson, R. I. (1999). Performance of Dyslexic Children on Cerebellar and Cognitive Tests. *J. Mot. Behav.,* 31(1), 68-78.

Fawcett, A. J. and Nicolson, R. I. (2004). Dyslexia: The role of the cerebellum. In: G. Reid and A. J. Fawcett (Eds.), *Dyslexia in context* (pp. 25-47). London: Whurr Publishers.

Fawcett, A. J., Nicolson, R. I. and Dean, P. (1996). Impaired performance of children with dyslexia on a range of cerebellar tasks. *Annals of Dyslexia,* 46, 259-283.

Fergusson, D. M. and Horwood, L. J. (1992). Attention deficit and reading achievement. *Journal of Child Psychology and Psychiatry,* 33, 375-385.

Fiez, J. A. and Raichle, M. E. (1997). Linguistic processing. *International Review of Neurobiology,* 41, 233-254.

Finch, A. J., Nicolson, R. I. and Fawcett, A. J. (2002). Evidence for a neuroanatomical difference within the olivo-cerebellar pathway of adults with dyslexia. *Cortex,* 38(4), 529-539.

Fisher, S. E. (2006). Tangled webs: tracing the connections between genes and cognition. *Cognition,* 101(2), 270-297.

Fisher, S. E., Francks, C., Marlow, A. J., MacPhie, I. L., Newbury, D. F., Cardon, L. R., Ishikawa-Brush, Y., Richardson, A. J., Talcott, J. B., Gayan, J., Olson, R. K., Pennington, B. F., Smith, S. D., DeFries, J. C., Stein, J. F., and Monaco, A. P. (2002). Independent genome-wide scans identify a chromosome 18 quantitative-trait locus influencing dyslexia. *Nat. Genet.,* 30(1), 86-91.

Fisher, S. E., Francks, C., McCracken, J. T., McGough, J. J., Marlow, A. J., MacPhie, I. L., Newbury, D. F., Crawford, L. R., Palmer, C. G., Woodward, J. A., Del'Homme, M., Cantwell, D. P., Nelson, S. F., Monaco, A. P., and Smalley, S. L. (2002). A genomewide scan for loci involved in attention-deficit/hyperactivity disorder. *Am. J. Hum. Genet.,* 70 (5), 1183-1196.

Francks, C., Paracchini, S., Smith, S. D., Richardson, A. J., Scerri, T. S., Cardon, L. R., Marlow, A. J., MacPhie, I. L., Walter, J., Pennington, B. F., Fisher, S. E., Olson, R. K., DeFries, J. C., Stein, J. F., and Monaco, A. P. (2004). A 77-kilobase region of chromosome 6p22.2 is associated with dyslexia in families from the United Kingdom and from the United States. *Am. J. Hum. Genet.,* 75(6), 1046-1058.

Friston, K. J. (2002). Statistics I: Experimental design and statistical parametric mapping. In: A. W. Toga and J. C. Mazziotta (Eds.), *Brain mapping: The methods* (Second ed., pp. 605-631). San Diego, US: Academic Press.

Friston, K. J., Frith, C. D., Liddle, P. F., and Frackowiak, R. S. (1993). Functional connectivity: the principal-component analysis of large (PET) data sets. *J. Cereb. Blood Flow Metab.,* 13(1), 5-14.

Frith, C. and Frith, U. (1996). A biological marker for dyslexia. *Nature,* 382, 19-20.

Frith, U. (1997). Brain, mind and behaviour in dyslexia. In: C. Hulme and M. Snowling (Eds.), *Dyslexia: biology, cognition and intervention* (pp. 1-19). London: Whurr Pulbishers Ltd.

Frith, U. (1999). Paradoxes in the definition of dyslexia. *Dyslexia. An International Journal of Research and Practice,* 5(4), 192–214.

Frost, S. J., Sandak, R., Mencl, W. E., Landi, N., Moore, D. L., Porta, G. D., Rueckl, J. G., Katz, L., and Pugh, K. R. (2008). Neurobiological and behavioural studies of skilled and impaired word reading. In: E. L. Grigorenko and A. J. Naples (Eds.), *Single-Word Reading* (pp. 355-376). New York: LEA.

Frye, R. E., Hasan, K., Xue, L., Strickland, D., Malmberg, B., Liederman, J., and Papanicolaou, A. (2008). Splenium microstructure is related to two dimensions of reading skill. *Neuroreport,* 19(16), 1627-1631.

Fulbright, R. K., Jenner, A. R., Mencl, W. E., Pugh, K. R., Shaywitz, B. A., Shaywitz, S. E., Frost, S. J., Skudlarski, P., Constable, R. T., Lacadie, C. M., Marchione, K. E., and Gore, J. C. (1999). The cerebellum's role in reading: a functional MR imaging study. *AJNR Am. J. Neuroradiol.,* 20(10), 1925-1930.

Gainotti, G., Miceli, G., Silveri, M. C., and Villa, G. (1982). Some anatomo-clinical aspects of phonemic and semantic comprehension disorders in aphasia. *Act. Neurol. Scand.,* 66, 652-665.

Galaburda, A. M. (2005). Dyslexia a molecular disorder of neuronal migration. *Annals of Dyslexia,* 55(2), 151-165.

Galaburda, A. M. and Kemper, T. L. (1979). Cytoarchitectonic abnormalities in developmental dyslexia: a case study. *Ann. Neurol.,* 6(2), 94-100.

Galaburda, A. M., LoTurco, J., Ramus, F., Fitch, R. H., and Rosen, G. D. (2006). From genes to behavior in developmental dyslexia. *Nat. Neurosci.* 9(10), 1213-1217.

Galaburda, A. M., Sherman, G. F., Rosen, G. D., Aboitiz, F., and Geschwind, N. (1985). Developmental dyslexia: four consecutive patients with cortical anomalies. *Ann. Neurol.,* 18(2), 222-233.

Gass, A. and Richards, T. L. (2013). Serial proton magnetic resonance spectroscopy of normal-appearing gray and white matter in MS. *Neurology,* 80(1), 17-18.

Geschwind, N. (1965). Disconnexion syndromes in animals and man. *Brain,* 88, 237–294.

Geyer, S. (2003). *The microstructural border between the motor and the cognitive domain in the human cerebral cortex.* Wien: Springer.

Geyer, S., Ledberg, A., Schleicher, A., Kinomura, S., Schormann, T., Burgel, U., Klingberg, T., Larsson, J., Zilles, K., and Roland, P. E. (1996). Two different areas within the primary motor cortex of man. *Nature,* 382(6594), 805-807.

Geyer, S., Schleicher, A. and Zilles, K. (1999). Areas 3a, 3b, and 1 of human primary somatosensory cortex. *Neuroimage,* 10(1), 63-83.

Geyer, S., Schormann, T., Mohlberg, H., and Zilles, K. (2000). Areas 3a, 3b, and 1 of human primary somatosensory cortex. Part 2. Spatial normalization to standard anatomical space. *Neuroimage,* 11(6 Pt 1), 684-696.

Gilger, J. W., Pennington, B. F. and DeFries, J. C. (1992). A twin study of the etiology of comorbidity: Attention deficit hyperactivity disorder and dyslexia. *Journal of American Academy of child and Adolescent Psychiatry,* 31, 343-348.

Gillebert, C. R., Mantini, D., Peeters, R., Dupont, P., and Vandenberghe, R. (2013). Cytoarchitectonic mapping of attentional selection and reorienting in parietal cortex. *Neuroimage,* 67, 257-272.

Gizewski, E. R., Timmann, D. and Forsting, M. (2004). Specific cerebellar activation during Braille reading in blind subjects. *Hum. Brain Mapp.,* 22(3), 229-235.

Glaser, D. E. (2006). Experimental design, *Talk given during Statistical Parametric Mapping Course.* Wellcome Department of Imaging Neuroscience, London.

Goswami, U. (2003). Why theories about developmental dyslexia require developmental designs. *Trends in Cognitive Sciences,* 7(12).

Gramsbergen, A. (2003). Clumsiness and disturbed cerebellar development: Insights from animal experiments, *Neural Plasticity,* 10(1-2), 129-140.

Habib, M. (2000). The neurological basis of developmental dyslexia: An overview and working hypothesis. *Brain,* 123, 2373-2399.

Hall, P. K. and Tomblin, J. B. (1978). A follow-up study of children with articulation and language disorders. *J. Speech Hear. Disord.,* 43(2), 227-241.

Hallgren, B. (1950). Specific dyslexia ('congenital word blindness'): a clinical and genetic study. *Acta Psychiatr. Neurol.,* 65, 2-289.

Hämäläinen, M. and Hari, R. (2002). Magnetoencephalographic characterisation of dynamic brain activation: Basic principles and methods of data collection and source analysis In: A. W. Toga and J. C. Mazziotta (Eds.), *Brain mapping: The methods* (pp. 227-253). San Diego, US: Academic Press.

Hanley, J. R. (1997). Reading and spelling impairments in undergraduate students with developmental dyslexia. *Journal of Research in Reading,* 20(1), 22-30.

Hannula-Jouppi, K., Kaminen-Ahola, N., Taipale, M., Eklund, R., Nopola-Hemmi, J., Kääriäinen, H., and Kere, J. (2005). The axon guidance receptor gene ROBO1 is a candidate gene for developmental dyslexia. *PLoS Genetics,* 1(4), e50.

Hansen, P. C., Stein, J. F., Orde, S. R., Winter, J. L., and Talcott, J. B. (2001). Are dyslexics' visual deficits limited to measures of dorsal stream function? *Neuroreport,* 12(7), 1527-1530.

Haslum, M. N. (1989). Predictors of dyslexia? *The Irish Journal of Psychology,* 10, 622-630.

Heim, S., Alter, K., Ischebeck, A. K., Amunts, K., Eickhoff, S. B., Mohlberg, H., Zilles, K., von Cramon, D. Y., and Friederici, A. D. (2005). The role of the left Brodmann's areas 44 and 45 in reading words and pseudowords. *Brain Res. Cogn. Brain Res.,* 25(3), 982-993.

Heim, S., Amunts, K., Hensel, T., Grande, M., Huber, W., Binkofski, F., and Eickhoff, S. B. (2012). The Role of Human Parietal Area 7A as a Link between Sequencing in Hand Actions and in Overt Speech Production. *Front Psychol.,* 3, 534.

Heim, S., Grande, M., Pape-Neumann, J., van Ermingen, M., Meffert, E., Grabowska, A., Huber, W., and Amunts, K. (2010). Interaction of phonological awareness and 'magnocellular' processing during normal and dyslexic reading: behavioural and fMRI investigations. *Dyslexia,* 16(3), 258-282.

Heim, S., Tschierse, J., Amunts, K., Wilms, M., Vossel, S., Willmes, K., Grabowska, A., and Huber, W. (2008). Cognitive subtypes of dyslexia. *Acta Neurobiol. Exp.* (Wars.), 68(1), 73-82.

Hickok, G. and Poeppel, D. (2004). Dorsal and ventral streams: a framework for understanding aspects of the functional anatomy of language. *Cognition,* 92(1-2), 67-99.

Hoeft, F., McCandliss, B. D., Black, J. M., Gantman, A., Zakerani, N., Hulme, C., Lyytinen, H., Whitfield-Gabrieli, S., Glover, G. H., Reiss, A. L., and Gabrieli, J. D. (2011). Neural systems predicting long-term outcome in dyslexia. *Proc. Natl. Acad. Sci. US,* 108(1), 361-366.

Hoeft, F., Meyler, A., Hernandez, A., Juel, C., Taylor-Hill, H., Martindale, J. L., McMillon, G., Kolchugina, G., Black, J. M., Faizi, A., Deutsch, G. K., Siok, W. T., Reiss, A. L., Whitfield-Gabrieli, S., and Gabrieli, J. D. (2007). Functional and morphometric brain dissociation between dyslexia and reading ability. *Proc. Natl. Acad. Sci. US,* 104(10), 4234-4239.

Holmes, G. (1939). The cerebellum of man. *Brain,* 62, 1-30.

Horwitz, B., Rumsey, J. M. and Donohue, B. C. (1998). Functional connectivity of the angular gyrus in normal reading and dyslexia. *Proc. Natl. Acad. Sci. US,* 95(15), 8939-8944.

Hulme, C. and Snowling, M. J. (2009). *Developmental disorders of language, learning and cognition.* Chichester, UK: Wiley-Blackwell.

Human Genome Project. (2011). Accessed on line http://www.ornl.gov/sci/techresources/Human_Genome/home.shtml on 02/08/11.

Igo, R. P., Jr., Chapman, N. H., Berninger, V. W., Matsushita, M., Brkanac, Z., Rothstein, J. H., Holzman, T., Nielsen, K., Raskind, W. H., and Wijsman, E. M. (2006). Genomewide scan for real-word reading subphenotypes of dyslexia: novel chromosome 13 locus and genetic complexity. *Am. J. Med. Genet. B Neuropsychiatr. Genet.,* 141B(1), 15-27.

International Dyslexia Association. (2009). International Dyslexia Association (2009). Official IDA definition of dyslexia. Accessed on line http://www.ne-ida.com/website/what_is_dyslexia on 05/08/09.

Ito, M. (1990). A new physiological concept on cerebellum. *Revue Neurol.,* 146, 564-569.

Ito, M. (2000). Mechanisms of motor learning in the cerebellum. *Brain Res.,* 886(1-2), 237-245.

Iversen, S., Berg, K., Ellertsen, B., and Tonnessen, F. E. (2005). Motor coordination difficulties in a municipality group and in a clinical sample of poor readers. *Dyslexia,* 11 (3), 217-231.

Ivry, R. B. (2003). Cerebellar involvement in clumsiness and other developmental disorders. *Neural Plasticity,* 10(1-2), 141-153.

Ivry, R. B. and Keele, S. W. (1989). Timing functions of the cerebellum. *Journal of Cognitive Neuroscience,* 1, 136-152.

Kaminen, N., Hannula-Jouppi, K., Kestila, M., Lahermo, P., Muller, K., Kaaranen, M., Myllyluoma, B., Voutilainen, A., Lyytinen, H., Nopola-Hemmi, J., and Kere, J. (2003). A genome scan for developmental dyslexia confirms linkage to chromosome 2p11 and suggests a new locus on 7q32. *J. Med. Genet.,* 40(5), 340-345.

Kaplan, B. J., Wilson, B. N., Dewey, D., and Crawford, S. G. (1998). DCD may not be a discrete disorder. *Human Movement Science,* 17, 471-490.

Karmiloff-Smith, A. (1998). Development itself is the key to understanding developmental disorders. *Trends in Cognitive Sciences,* 2(10), 389-398.

Kashiwagi, M., Iwaki, S., Narumi, Y., Tamai, H., and Suzuki, S. (2009). Parietal dysfunction in developmental coordination disorder: a functional MRI study. *Neuroreport,* 20(15), 1319-1324.

Keller, T. A. and Just, M. A. (2009). Altering cortical connectivity: remediation-induced changes in the white matter of poor readers. *Neuron,* 64(5), 624-631.

Kertesz, A., Harlock, W. and Coates, R. (1979). Computer tomographic localization, lesion size, and prognosis in aphasia and non-verbal impairment. *Brain Lang.* 8, 34-50.

Kiernan, J. A. (2009). *The human nervous system. An anatomical viewpoint* (9th ed.). Baltimore, US: Lippincott Williams and Wilkins.

Klingberg, T., Hedehus, M., Temple, E., Salz, T., Gabrieli, J. D., Moseley, M. E., and Poldrack, R. A. (2000). Microstructure of temporo-parietal white matter as a basis for reading ability: evidence from diffusion tensor magnetic resonance imaging. *Neuron,* 25 (2), 493-500.

Klintsova, A. Y., Goodlett, C. R. and Greenough, W. T. (2000). Therapeutic motor training ameliorates cerebellar effects of postnatal binge alcohol. *Neurotoxicology and Teratology,* 22, 125-132.

Knecht, S., Drager, B., Deppe, M., Bobe, L., Lohmann, H., Floel, A., Ringelstein, E. B., and Henningsen, H. (2000). Handedness and hemispheric language dominance in healthy humans. *Brain,* 123 Pt 12, 2512-2518.

Kronbichler, M., Wimmer, H., Staffen, W., Hutzler, F., Mair, A., and Ladurner, G. (2008). Developmental dyslexia: gray matter abnormalities in the occipitotemporal cortex. *Hum. Brain Mapp.,* 29(5), 613-625.

Kurth, F., Eickhoff, S. B., Schleicher, A., Hoemke, L., Zilles, K., and Amunts, K. (2009). Cytoarchitecture and Probabilistic Maps of the Human Posterior Insular Cortex. *Cereb. Cortex.*

Laing, E., Hulme, C., Grant, J., and Karmiloff-Smith, A. (2001). Learning to read in Williams syndrome: looking beneath the surface of atypical reading development. *J. Child Psychol. Psychiatry,* 42(6), 729-739.

Laycock, S. K., Wilkinson, I. D., Wallis, L. I., Darwent, G., Wonders, S. H., Fawcett, A. J., Griffiths, P. D., and Nicolson, R. I. (2008). Cerebellar volume and cerebellar metabolic characteristics in adults with dyslexia. *Ann. N Y Acad. Sci.,* 1145, 222-236.

Leiner, H. C., Leiner, A. L. and Dow, R. S. (1993). Cognitive and language functions of the human cerebellum. *TINS,* 16, 444-447.

Liederman, J., McGraw Fisher, J., Schulz, M., Maxwell, C., Theoret, H., and Pascual-Leone, A. (2003). The role of motion direction selective extrastriate regions in reading: a transcranial magnetic stimulation study. *Brain Lang.,* 85(1), 140-155.

Light, J. G., Pennington, B. F., Gilger, J. W., and DeFries, J. C. (1995). Reading disability and hyperactivity disorder: evidence for a common genetic etiology. *Developmental Neuropsychology,* 11, 323–335.

Londin, E. R., Meng, H. and Gruen, J. R. (2003). A transcription map of the 6p22.3 reading disability locus identifying candidate genes. *BMC Genomics,* 4(1), 25.

Loo, S. K., Fisher, S. E., Francks, C., Ogdie, M. N., MacPhie, I. L., Yang, M., McCracken, J. T., McGough, J. J., Nelson, S. F., Monaco, A. P., and Smalley, S. L. (2004). Genome-wide scan of reading ability in affected sibling pairs with attention-deficit/hyperactivity disorder: unique and shared genetic effects. *Mol. Psychiatry,* 9(5), 485-493.

Lovegrove, W. J., Martin, F., Bowling, A., Blackwood, M., Badcock, D., and Paxton, S. (1982). Contrast sensitivity functions and specific reading disability. *Neuropsychologia,* 20, 309–315.

Lundberg, I. and Hoien, T. (2001). Dyslexia and phonology. In: A. Fawcett (Ed.), *Dyslexia: Theory and good practice* (pp. 109–123). London: Whurr Publishers.

Lurito, J. T., Kareken, D. A., Dzemidzic, M., Lowe, M. J., Radnovich, A., Staser, J., Phillips, M. D., Wang, Y., and Mathews, V. P. (2000). Functional MRI of covert object naming. *NemoImage,* 11(5), S285.

MacDermot, K. D., Bonora, E., Sykes, N., Coupe, A. M., Lai, C. S., Vernes, S. C., Vargha-Khadem, F., McKenzie, F., Smith, R. L., Monaco, A. P., and Fisher, S. E. (2005). Identification of FOXP2 truncation as a novel cause of developmental speech and language deficits. *Am. J. Hum. Genet.,* 76(6), 1074-1080.

Maisog, J. M., Einbinder, E. R., Flowers, D. L., Turkeltaub, P. E., and Eden, G. F. (2008). A meta-analysis of functional neuroimaging studies of dyslexia. *Ann. N Y Acad. Sci.,* 1145, 237-259.

Malikovic, A., Amunts, K., Schleicher, A., Mohlberg, H., Eickhoff, S. B., Wilms, M., Palomero-Gallagher, N., Armstrong, E., and Zilles, K. (2007). Cytoarchitectonic analysis of the human extrastriate cortex in the region of V5/MT+: a probabilistic, stereotaxic map of area hOc5. *Cereb. Cortex,* 17(3), 562-574.

Manto, M., Gruol, D. L., Schmahmann, J. D., Koibuchi, N., and Rossi, F. (Eds.). (2013). *Handbook of the cerebellum and cerebellar disorders*. Dordrecht: Springer.

Marien, P., Engelborghs, S., Fabbro, F., and De Deyn, P. P. (2001). The lateralized linguistic cerebellum: a review and a new hypothesis. *Brain Lang.,* 79(3), 580-600.

Marien, P., Wackenier, P., De Surgeloose, D., De Deyn, P. P., and Verhoeven, J. (2010). Developmental coordination disorder: disruption of the cerebello-cerebral network evidenced by SPECT. *Cerebellum,* 9(3), 405-410.

Mathiak, K. and Fallgatter, A. J. (2005). Combining magnetoencephalography and functional magnetic resonance imaging. *International Review of Neurobiology,* 68, 122-148.

Matthews, P. M. (2001). An introduction to functional magnetic resonance imaging of the brain. In: P. Jezzard and P. M. Matthews and S. M. Smith (Eds.), *Functional MRI. An introduction to methods.* (pp. 3-34). Oxford, UK: Oxford University Press.

Maudsley, A. A. (2002). Magnetic resonance spectroscopic imaging. In: A. W. Toga and J. C. Mazziotta (Eds.), *Brain mapping: The methods* (Second ed.). San Diego, US: Academic Press.

McCall, R. B. (1977). Childhood IQ's as Predictors of Adult Educational and Occupational Status. *Science,* 197(4302), 482-483.

McCrory, E. J., Mechelli, A., Frith, U., and Price, C. J. (2005). More than words: a common neural basis for reading and naming deficits in developmental dyslexia? *Brain,* 128(Pt 2), 261-267.

McDermott, K. B., Petersen, S. E., Watson, J. M., and Ojemann, J. G. (2003). A procedure for identifying regions preferentially activated by attention to semantic and phonological relations using functional magnetic resonance imaging. *Neuropsychologia,* 41(3), 293-303.

McPhillips, M. and Sheehy, N. (2004). Prevalence of persistent primary reflexes and motor problems in children with reading difficulties. *Dyslexia,* 10(4), 316-338.

Meng, H., Smith, S. D., Hager, K., Held, M., Liu, J., Olson, R. K., Pennington, B. F., DeFries, J. C., Gelernter, J., O'Reilly-Pol, T., Somlo, S., Skudlarski, P., Shaywitz, S. E., Shaywitz, B. A., Marchione, K., Wang, Y., Paramasivam, M., LoTurcok, J. J., Pagel, G. P., and Gruen, J. R. (2005). DCDC2 is associated with reading disability and modulates neuronal development in the brain. *Proceedings of the National Academy of Science of the US,* 102(47), 17053-17058.

Menghini, D., Finzi, A., Benassi, M., Bolzani, R., Facoetti, A., Giovagnoli, S., Ruffino, M., and Vicari, S. (2010). Different underlying neurocognitive deficits in developmental dyslexia: a comparative study. *Neuropsychologia,* 48(4), 863-872.

Mesulam, M. M. (1990). Large scale neurocognitive networks and distributed processing for attention, language and memory. *Annals of Neurology,* 28, 597-613.

Meyer-Lindenberg, A., Mervis, C. B. and Berman, K. F. (2006). Neural mechanisms in Williams syndrome: a unique window to genetic influences on cognition and behaviour. *Nat. Rev. Neurosci.,* 7(5), 380-393.

Miles, T. R. (1993). *Dyslexia: The pattern of difficulties* (2nd ed.). London: Whurr.

Milne, R. D., Syngeniotis, A., Jackson, G., and Corballis, M. C. (2002). Mixed lateralization of phonological assembly in developmental dyslexia. *Neurocase,* 8(3), 205-209.

Moore, C. J. and Price, C. J. (1999). Three distinct ventral occipitotemporal regions for reading and object naming. *Neuroimage,* 10, 181-192.

Morosan, P., Schleicher, A., Amunts, K., and Zilles, K. (2005). Multimodal architectonic mapping of human superior temporal gyrus. *Anatomy and Embryology,* 210, 401–406.

Morton, J. and Frith, U. (1995). Causal modeling: A structural approach to developmental psycho pathology. In: D. Cicchetti and D. J. Cohen (Eds.), *Manual of Developmental Psychopathology* (pp. 357-390). New York: Wiley.

Newbury, D. F., Paracchini, S., Scerri, T. S., Winchester, L., Addis, L., Richardson, A. J., Walter, J., Stein, J. F., Talcott, J. B., and Monaco, A. P. (2011). Investigation of dyslexia and SLI risk variants in reading- and language-impaired subjects. *Behav. Genet.,* 41(1), 90-104.

Newsome, W. T. and Pare, E. B. (1988). A selective impairment of motion processing following lesions of the middle temporal visual area (MT). *Journal of Neuroscience,* 8, 2201–2211.

Nicolson, R. I., Daum, I., Schugens, M. M., Fawcett, A. J., and Schulz, A. (2002). Eyeblink conditioning indicates cerebellar abnormality in dyslexia. *Exp. Brain Res.,* 143(1), 42-50.

Nicolson, R. I. and Fawcett, A. J. (1990). Automaticity: a new framework for dyslexia research? *Cognition,* 35(2), 159-182.

Nicolson, R. I. and Fawcett, A. J. (2008). *Dyslexia, learning, and the brain.* Cambridge, Massachusetts; London, England: MIT Press.

Nicolson, R. I., Fawcett, A. J., Berry, E. L., Jenkins, I. H., Dean, P., and Brooks, D. J. (1999). Association of abnormal cerebellar activation with motor learning difficulties in dyslexic adults. *Lancet,* 353(9165), 1662-1667.

Nicolson, R. I., Fawcett, A. J. and Dean, P. (2001). Developmental dyslexia: the cerebellar deficit hypothesis. *Trends Neurosci.,* 24(9), 508-511.

Niogi, S. N. and McCandliss, B. D. (2006). Left lateralized white matter microstructure accounts for individual differences in reading ability and disability. *Neuropsychologia,* 44 (11), 2178-2188.

Nopola-Hemmi, J., Myllyluoma, B., Haltia, T., Taipale, M., Ollikainen, V., Ahonen, T., Voutilainen, A., Kere, J., and Widen, E. (2001). A dominant gene for developmental dyslexia on chromosome 3. *J. Med. Genet.,* 38(10), 658-664.

Nopoulos, P. C., Ceilley, J. W., Gailis, E. A., and Andreasen, N. C. (1999). An MRI study of cerebellar vermis morphology in patients with schizophrenia: Evidence in support of the cognitive dysmetria concept. *Biol. Psychiatry* 46, 703-711.

O'Hare, A. and Khalid, S. (2002). The association of abnormal cerebellar function in children with developmental coordination disorder and reading difficulties. *Dyslexia,* 8(4), 234-248.

Odegard, T. N., Farris, E. A., Ring, J., McColl, R., and Black, J. (2009). Brain connectivity in non-reading impaired children and children diagnosed with developmental dyslexia. *Neuropsychologia,* 47(8-9), 1972-1977.

Ogdie, M. N., Macphie, I. L., Minassian, S. L., Yang, M., Fisher, S. E., Francks, C., Cantor, R. M., McCracken, J. T., McGough, J. J., Nelson, S. F., Monaco, A. P., and Smalley, S. L. (2003). A genomewide scan for attention-deficit/hyperactivity disorder in an extended sample: suggestive linkage on 17p11. *Am. J. Hum. Genet.,* 72(5), 1268-1279.

Olson, R., Forsberg, H., Wise, B., and Rack, J. (1994). Measurement of word recognition, orthographic, and phonological skills. In: G. R. Lyon (Ed.), *Frames of reference for the assessment of learning disabilities: New views on measurement issues* (pp. 243-277). Baltimore: Paul H. Brookes.

Olson, R., Wise, B., Conners, F., Rack, J., and Fulker, D. (1989). Specific deficits in component reading and language skills: Genetic and environmental influences. *Journal of Learning Disabilities,* 22, 339-349.

Olson, R. K., Datta, H. J. G. and DeFries, J. C. (1999). A behaviour-genetic analysis of reading disabilities and component processes. In: R. M. Klein and P. McMullen (Eds.), *Converging methods for understanding reading and dyslexia* (pp. 133-152). Cambridge, MA: MIT Press.

Pagnamenta, A. T., Bacchelli, E., de Jonge, M. V., Mirza, G., Scerri, T. S., Minopoli, F., Chiocchetti, A., Ludwig, K. U., Hoffmann, P., Paracchini, S., Lowy, E., Harold, D. H., Chapman, J. A., Klauck, S. M., Poustka, F., Houben, R. H., Staal, W. G., Ophoff, R. A., O'Donovan, M. C., Williams, J., Nothen, M. M., Schulte-Korne, G., Deloukas, P., Ragoussis, J., Bailey, A. J., Maestrini, E., and Monaco, A. P. (2010). Characterization of a family with rare deletions in CNTNAP5 and DOCK4 suggests novel risk loci for autism and dyslexia. *Biol. Psychiatry,* 68(4), 320-328.

Paracchini, S., Thomas, A., Castro, S., Lai, C., Paramasivam, M., Wang, Y., Keating, B. J., Taylor, J. M., Hacking, D. F., Scerri, T., Francks, C., Richardson, A. J., Wade-Martins, R., Stein, J. F., Knight, J. C., Copp, A. J., LoTurco, J., and Monaco, A. P. (2006). The chromosome 6p22 haplotype associated with dyslexia reduces the expression of KIAA0319, a novel gene involved in neuronal migration. *Human Molecular Genetics,* 15 (10), 1659–1666.

Pascual-Leone, A. and Walsh, V. (2002). Transcranial magnetic stimulation. In: A. W. Toga and J. C. Mazziotta (Eds.), *Brain mapping: The methods* (Second ed.). San Diego, US: Academic Press.

Paulesu, E., Demonet, J. F., Fazio, F., McCrory, E., Chanoine, V., Brunswick, N., Cappa, S. F., Cossu, G., Habib, M., Frith, C. D., and Frith, U. (2001). Dyslexia: cultural diversity and biological unity. *Science,* 291(5511), 2165-2167.

Paulesu, E., Frith, C. D. and Frackowiak, R. S. J. (1993). The neural correlates of the verbal component of working memory. *Nature,* 362, 342-345.

Paulesu, E., Frith, U., Snowling, M., Gallagher, A., Morton, J., Frackowiak, R. S., and Frith, C. D. (1996). Is developmental dyslexia a disconnection syndrome? Evidence from PET scanning. *Brain,* 119 (Pt 1), 143-157.

Paulesu, E., McCrory, E., Fazio, F., Menoncello, L., Brunswick, N., Cappa, S. F., Cotelli, M., Cossu, G., Corte, F., Lorusso, M., Pesenti, S., Gallagher, A., Perani, D., Price, C., Frith, C. D., and Frith, U. (2000). A cultural effect on brain function. *Nat. Neurosci.,* 3(1), 91-96.

Pennington, B. F. (2006). From single to multiple deficit models of developmental disorders. *Cognition,* 101, 385-413.

Pennington, B. F. (2011). *Using genetics and neuropsychology to understand dyslexia and its comorbidities.* Paper presented at the 8th BDA International Conference, Harrogate, UK, June.

Pennington, B. F. and Bishop, D. V. (2009). Relations among speech, language, and reading disorders. *Annu. Rev. Psychol.,* 60, 283-306.

Perfetti, C. A. and Bolger, D. J. (2004). The brain might read that way. *Scientific Studies of Reading,* 8(3), 293-304.

Pernet, C. R., Poline, J. B., Demonet, J. F., and Rousselet, G. A. (2009). Brain classification reveals the right cerebellum as the best biomarker of dyslexia. *BMC Neurosci.,* 10, 67.

Peter, B., Raskind, W. H., Matsushita, M., Lisowski, M., Vu, T., Berninger, V. W., Wijsman, E. M., and Brkanac, Z. (2011). Replication of CNTNAP2 association with nonword repetition and support for FOXP2 association with timed reading and motor activities in a dyslexia family sample. *J. Neurodev. Disord.,* 3(1), 39-49.

Pinel, P., Fauchereau, F., Moreno, A., Barbot, A., Lathrop, M., Zelenika, D., Le Bihan, D., Poline, J. B., Bourgeron, T., and Dehaene, S. (2012). Genetic variants of FOXP2 and KIAA0319/TTRAP/THEM2 locus are associated with altered brain activation in distinct language-related regions. *J. Neurosci.,* 32(3), 817-825.

Plomin, R., DeFries, J. C., McClearn, G. E., and McGuffin, P. (2008). *Behavioural genetics* (5th ed.). New York: Worth Publishers.

Poelmans, G., Buitelaar, J. K., Pauls, D. L., and Franke, B. (2011). A theoretical molecular network for dyslexia: integrating available genetic findings. *Mol. Psychiatry,* 16(4), 365-382.

Poelmans, G., Engelen, J. J., Van Lent-Albrechts, J., Smeets, H. J., Schoenmakers, E., Franke, B., Buitelaar, J. K., Wuisman-Frerker, M., Erens, W., Steyaert, J., and Schrander-Stumpel, C. (2009). Identification of novel dyslexia candidate genes through the analysis of a chromosomal deletion. *Am. J. Med. Genet. B Neuropsychiatr. Genet.,* 150B(1), 140-147.

Poeppel, D., Idsardi, W. J. and Wassenhove, V. (2009). Speech perception at the interface of neurobiology and linguistic. In: B. C. Moore and L. K. Tyler and W. D. Marslen-Wilson (Eds.), *The perception of speech* (pp. 249-274). Oxford: Oxford University Press.

Poldrack, R. A., Fletcher, P. C., Henson, R. N., Worsley, K. J., Brett, M., and Nichols, T. E. (2008). Guidelines for reporting an fMRI study. *Neuroimage,* 40(2), 409-414.

Poldrack, R. A., Mumford, J. A. and Nichols, T. E. (2011). *Handbook of functional MRI data analysis*. Cambridge: Cambridge University Press.

Portwood, M. (2000). *Understanding developmental dyspraxia*. London: David Fulton Publishers.

Price, C. J. (2000). The anatomy of language: contributions from functional neuroimaging. *J. Anat.,* 197 Pt 3, 335-359.

Price, C. J. (2010). The anatomy of language: a review of 100 fMRI studies published in 2009. *Ann. N Y Acad. Sci.,* 1191, 62-88.

Price, C. J. and Devlin, J. T. (2003). The myth of the visual word form area. *Neuroimage,* 19 (3), 473-481.

Price, C. J. and Mechelli, A. (2005). Reading and reading disturbance. *Current Opinion in Neurobiology,* 15, 231-238.

Price, C. J., Moore, C. J. and Frackowiak, R. S. (1996). The Effect of Varying Stimulus Rate and Duration on Brain Activity during Reading. *Neuroimage,* 3, 40-52.

Price, C. J., Moore, C. J., Humphreys, G. W., and Wise, R. J. S. (1997). Segregating semantic from phonological processes during reading. *Journal of Cognitive neuroscience,* 6, 727-733.

Price, C. J., Wise, R. J. and Frackowiak, R. S. (1996). Demonstrating the implicit processing of visually presented words and pseudowords. *Cereb. Cortex,* 6(1), 62-70.

Pugh, K. R. (2006). *Neuroimaging studies of skilled reading and reading disability.* Paper presented at the 57th Annual IDA Conference, Indianapolis, US.

Pugh, K. R., Frost, S. J., Rothman, D. L., Hoeft, F., Del Tufo, S. N., Mason, G. F., Molfese, P. J., Mencl, W. E., Grigorenko, E. L., Landi, N., Preston, J. L., Jacobsen, L., Seidenberg, M. S., and Fulbright, R. K. (2014). Glutamate and choline levels predict individual differences in reading ability in emergent readers. *J. Neurosci.,* 34(11), 4082-4089.

Pugh, K. R., Mencl, W. E., Jenner, A. R., Katz, L., Frost, S. J., Lee, J. R., Shaywitz, S. E., and Shaywitz, B. A. (2000). Functional neuroimaging studies of reading and reading disability (developmental dyslexia). *Ment. Retard. Dev. Disabil. Res. Rev.,* 6(3), 207-213.

Pugh, K. R., Mencl, W. E., Shaywitz, B. A., Shaywitz, S. E., Fulbright, R. K., Constable, R. T., Skudlarski, P., Marchione, K. E., Jenner, A. R., Fletcher, J. M., Liberman, A. M., Shankweiler, D. P., Katz, L., Lacadie, C., and Gore, J. C. (2000). The angular gyrus in developmental dyslexia: task-specific differences in functional connectivity within posterior cortex. *Psychol. Sci.,* 11(1), 51-56.

Purpura, K., Kaplan, E. and Shapley, R. M. (1988). Background light and the contrast gain of primate P and M retinal ganglion cells. *Proc. Natl. Acad. Sci. US* 85, 4534–4537.

Rack, J. (1997). Issues in the assessment of developmental dyslexia in adults: Theoretical and applied perspectives. *Journal of Research in Reading,* 20, 66-76.

Rack, J. P., Snowling, M. J. and Olson, R. K. (1992). The nonword reading deficit in developmental dyslexia: A review. *Reading Research Quarterly,* 27(1), 29–53.

Rae, C., Harasty, J. A., Dzendrowskyj, T. E., Talcott, J. B., Simpson, J. M., Blamire, A. M., Dixon, R. M., Lee, M. A., Thompson, C. H., Styles, P., Richardson, A. J., and Stein, J. F. (2002). Cerebellar morphology in developmental dyslexia. *Neuropsychologia,* 40(8), 1285-1292.

Rae, C., Lee, M. A., Dixon, R. M., Blamire, A. M., Thompson, C. H., Styles, P., Talcott, J., Richardson, A. J., and Stein, J. F. (1998). Metabolic abnormalities in developmental dyslexia detected by 1H magnetic resonance spectroscopy. *Lancet,* 351(9119), 1849-1852.

Ramus, F. (2004). Should neuroconstructivism guide developmental research? *Trends Cogn. Sci.,* 8(3), 100-101.

Ramus, F., Rosen, S., Dakin, S. C., Day, B. L., Castellote, J. M., White, S., and Frith, U. (2003). Theories of developmental dyslexia: insights from a multiple case study of dyslexic adults. *Brain,* 126(Pt 4), 841-865.

Ramus, F. and Szenkovits, G. (2008). What phonological deficit? *The Quarterly Journal of Experimental Psychology,* 61(1), 129–141.

Rayner, K. and Pollatsek, A. (1989). *The psychology of reading.* Hillsdale, New Jersey: LEA.

Reid, A. A. and Hansen, P. (2013). University students with dyslexia: their deficits, strengths, cognitive styles and learning strategies. *Manuscript in preparation.*

Reid, A. A., Szczerbinski, M., Iskierka-Kasperek, E., and Hansen, P. (2007). Cognitive profiles of adult developmental dyslexics: Theoretical implications. *Dyslexia,* 13, 1-24.

Riccio, C. A. and Hynd, G. W. (1993). Developmental language disorders in children: Relationship with learning disability and attention deficit hyperactivity disorder. *School Psychology Review,* 22, 696-709.

Richards, T., Stevenson, J., Crouch, J., Johnson, L. C., Maravilla, K., Stock, P., Abbott, R., and Berninger, V. (2008). Tract-based spatial statistics of diffusion tensor imaging in adults with dyslexia. *AJNR Am. J. Neuroradiol.,* 29(6), 1134-1139.

Rimrodt, S. L., Peterson, D. J., Denckla, M. B., Kaufmann, W. E., and Cutting, L. E. (2010). White matter microstructural differences linked to left perisylvian language network in children with dyslexia. *Cortex,* 46(6), 739-749.

Robbins, T. W. and Stavroula, K. (2011). Uncovering the genetic underpinnings of cognition. *Trends in Cognitive Sciences,* 15(9), 375-377.

Rochelle, K. S. H. and Talcott, J. B. (2006). Impaired balance in developmental dyslexia? A meta-analysis of the contending evidence. *Journal of Child Psychology and Psychiatry* 47(11), 1159–1166.

Rochelle, K. S. H., Witton, C. and Talcott, J. B. (2009). Symptoms of hyperactivity and inattention can mediate deficits of postural stability in developmental dyslexia. *Experimental Brain Research,* 192, 627-633.

Romero, L., Walsh, V. and Papagno, C. (2006). The neural correlates of phonological short-term memory: a repetitive transcranial magnetic stimulation study. *J. Cogn. Neurosci.,* 18 (7), 1147-1155.

Rosen, G. D., Bai, J., Wang, Y., Fiondella, C. G., Threlkeld, S. W., LoTurco, J. J., and Galaburda, A. M. (2007). Disruption of neuronal migration by RNAi of Dyx1c1 results in neocortical and hippocampal malformations. *Cerebral Cortex,* 17, 2562-2572.

Rottschy, C., Eickhoff, S. B., Schleicher, A., Mohlberg, H., Kujovic, M., Zilles, K., and Amunts, K. (2007). Ventral visual cortex in humans: cytoarchitectonic mapping of two extrastriate areas. *Hum. Brain Mapp.,* 28(10), 1045-1059.

Rumsey, J. M., Nace, K., Donohue, B., Wise, D., Maisog, J. M., and Andreason, P. (1997). A positron emission tomographic study of impaired word recognition and phonological processing in dyslexic men. *Arch. Neurol.,* 54(5), 562-573.

Rutter, M., Caspi, A., Fergusson, D., Horwood, L. J., Goodman, R., Maughan, B., Moffitt, T. E., Meltzer, H., and Carroll, J. (2004). Sex differences in developmental reading disability: new findings from 4 epidemiological studies. *Jama,* 291(16), 2007-2012.

Salmelin, R. and Helenius, P. (2004). Functional neuroanatomy of impaired reading in dyslexia. *Scientific Studies of Reading,* 8(3), 257-272.

Salmelin, R., Service, E., Kiesila, P., Uutela, K., and Salonen, O. (1996). Impaired visual word processing in dyslexia revealed with magnetoencephalography. *Ann. Neurol.,* 40(2), 157-162.

Samar, V. J. and Parasnis, I. (2005). Dorsal stream deficits suggest hidden dyslexia among deaf poor readers: Correlated evidence from reduced perceptual speed and elevated coherent motion detection thresholds. *Brain and Cognition,* 58(3), 300–311.

Sandak, R., Mencl, W. E., Frost, S. J., and Pugh, K. R. (2004). The neurobiological basis of skilled and impaired reading: Recent findings and new directions. *Scientific Studies of Reading,* 8(3), 273-292.

Scarborough, H. S. and Dobrich, W. (1990). Development of children with early language delay. *J. Speech Hear. Res.,* 33(1), 70-83.

Scerri, T. S., Darki, F., Newbury, D. F., Whitehouse, A. J., Peyrard-Janvid, M., Matsson, H., Ang, Q. W., Pennell, C. E., Ring, S., Stein, J., Morris, A. P., Monaco, A. P., Kere, J., Talcott, J. B., Klingberg, T., and Paracchini, S. (2012). The dyslexia candidate locus on 2p12 is associated with general cognitive ability and white matter structure. *PLoS One,* 7 (11), e50321.

Scerri, T. S., Morris, A. P., Buckingham, L. L., Newbury, D. F., Miller, L. L., Monaco, A. P., Bishop, D. V., and Paracchini, S. (2011). DCDC2, KIAA0319 and CMIP are associated with reading-related traits. *Biol. Psychiatry,* 70(3), 237-245.

Scheperjans, F., Eickhoff, S. B., Homke, L., Mohlberg, H., Hermann, K., Amunts, K., and Zilles, K. (2008). Probabilistic maps, morphometry, and variability of cytoarchitectonic areas in the human superior parietal cortex. *Cereb. Cortex,* 18(9), 2141-2157.

Scheperjans, F., Hermann, K., Eickhoff, S. B., Amunts, K., Schleicher, A., and Zilles, K. (2008). Observer-independent cytoarchitectonic mapping of the human superior parietal cortex. *Cereb. Cortex,* 18(4), 846-867.

Schlang, G. (2001). The brain of musicians. *Annals of the New York Academy of Sciences,* 930, 281-299.

Schmahmann, J. D. (Ed.). (1997). *The Cerebellum and cognition* (Vol. 41). San Diego, California: Academic Press.

Seines, O. A., Knopman, D. S., Niccum, N., and Rubens, A. B. (1985). The critical role of Wernicke's area in sentence repetition. *Ann. Neurol.,* 17, 549-557.

Semrud-Clikeman, M., Biederman, J., Sprich-Buckminster, S., Lehman, B. K., Faraone, S. V., and Norman, D. (1992). Comorbidity between attention defcit hyperactivity disorder and learning disability: A review and report in a clinically referred sample. *Journal of Amer. Academy of Child and Adolescent Psychiatry,* 31(3), 439-448.

Shanahan, M. A., Pennington, B. F., Yerys, B. E., Scott, A., Boada, R., Willcutt, E. G., Olson, R. K., and DeFries, J. C. (2006). Processing speed deficits in attention deficit/ hyperactivity disorder and reading disability. *J. Abnorm. Child Psychol.,* 34(5), 585-602.

Shaywitz, B. A., Shaywitz, S. E., Blachman, B. A., Pugh, K. R., Fulbright, R. K., Skudlarski, P., Mencl, W. E., Constable, R. T., Holahan, J. M., Marchione, K. E., Fletcher, J. M., Lyon, G. R., and Gore, J. C. (2004). Development of left occipitotemporal systems for skilled reading in children after a phonologically- based intervention. *Biol. Psychiatry,* 55 (9), 926-933.

Shaywitz, S. E. (1998). Current concepts: Dyslexia. *N. Engl. J. Med.,* 338, 307–312.

Shaywitz, S. E., Shaywitz, B. A., Fulbright, R. K., Skudlarski, P., Mencl, W. E., Constable, R. T., Pugh, K. R., Holahan, J. M., Marchione, K. E., Fletcher, J. M., Lyon, G. R., and Gore, J. C. (2003). Neural systems for compensation and persistence: young adult outcome of childhood reading disability. *Biol. Psychiatry,* 54(1), 25-33.

Shaywitz, S. E., Shaywitz, B. A., Pugh, K. R., Fulbright, R. K., Constable, R. T., Mencl, W. E., Shankweiler, D. P., Liberman, A. M., Skudlarski, P., Fletcher, J. M., Katz, L., Marchione, K. E., Lacadie, C., Gatenby, C., and Gore, J. C. (1998). Functional disruption in the organization of the brain for reading in dyslexia. *Proc. Natl. Acad. Sci. US,* 95(5), 2636-2641.

Simos, P. G., Fletcher, J. M., Bergman, E., Breier, J. I., Foorman, B. R., Castillo, E. M., Davis, R. N., Fitzgerald, M., and Papanicolaou, A. C. (2002). Dyslexia-specific brain activation profile becomes normal following successful remedial training. *Neurology,* 58 (8), 1203-1213.

Skottun, B. C. (2000). The magnocellular deficit theory of dyslexia: The evidence from contrast sensitivity. *Vision Research,* 40, 111–127.

Smalley, S. L. (1997). Genetic influences in childhood-onset psychiatric disorders: autism and attention-deficit/hyperactivity disorder. *Am. J. Hum. Genet.,* 60(6), 1276-1282.

Smalley, S. L., Kustanovich, V., Minassian, S. L., Stone, J. L., Ogdie, M. N., McGough, J. J., McCracken, J. T., MacPhie, I. L., Francks, C., Fisher, S. E., Cantor, R. M., Monaco, A. P., and Nelson, S. F. (2002). Genetic linkage of attention-deficit/hyperactivity disorder on chromosome 16p13, in a region implicated in autism. *Am. J. Hum. Genet.,* 71(4), 959-963.

Snell, R. S. (2001). *Clinical neuroanatomy for medical students* (5th ed.). Baltimore, US: Lippincott Williams and Wilkins.

Snowling, M., Bishop, D. V. and Stothard, S. E. (2000). Is preschool language impairment a risk factor for dyslexia in adolescence? *J. Child Psychol. Psychiatry,* 41(5), 587-600.

Snowling, M. J. (2000). *Dyslexia* (2nd ed.). Oxford: Blackwell.

Snowling, M. J. (2008). Specific disorders and broader phenotypes: The case of dyslexia. *The Quarterly Journal of Experimental Psychology,* 61(1), 142–156.

Snowling, M. J. (1980). The development of grapheme-phoneme correspondence in normal and dyslexic readers. *Journal of Experimental Child Psychology,* 29(2), 294–305.

Snowling, M. J. and Caravolas, M. (2007). Developmental dyslexia. In: M. G. Gaskell (Ed.), *The Oxford Handbook of Psycholinguistics* (pp. 667-683). Oxford: Oxford University Press.

Stein, J. (2001). The magnocellular theory of developmental dyslexia. *Dyslexia,* 7(1), 12-36.

Stein, J. (2003). Visual motion sensitivity and reading. *Neuropsychologia,* 41, 1785–1793.

Stein, J. and Kapoula, Z. (2012). *Visual Aspects of Dyslexia* (Kindle Edition ed.). Oxford: Oxford University Press.

Stein, J. and Talcott, J. (1999). Impaired neuronal timing in developmental dyslexia - the magnocellular hypothesis. *Dyslexia. An International Journal of Research and Practice,* 5, 59–77.

Stein, J., Talcott, J. and Witton, C. (2001). The sensorimotor basis of developmental dyslexia. In: A. J. Fawcett (Ed.), *Dyslexia: Theory and good practice* (pp. 65-88). London: Whurr Publishers.

Stein, J. and Walsh, V. (1997). To see but not to read; the magnocellular theory of dyslexia. *Trends Neurosci.,* 20(4), 147-152.

Stein, J. F. and Glickstein, M. (1992). Role of cerebellum in visual guidance of movement. *Physiological Reviews* 72, 972-1017.

Steinbrink, C., Vogt, K., Kastrup, A., Muller, H. P., Juengling, F. D., Kassubek, J., and Riecker, A. (2008). The contribution of white and gray matter differences to developmental dyslexia: insights from DTI and VBM at 3.0 T. *Neuropsychologia,* 46 (13), 3170-3178.

Stevenson, J., Pennington, B. F., Gilger, J. W., DeFries, J. C., and Gillis, J. J. (2006). Hyperactivity and spelling disability: Testing for shared genetic aetiology. *Journal of Child Psychology and Psychiatry,* 34(7), 1137-1152.

Stoeckel, C., Gough, P. M., Watkins, K. E., and Devlin, J. T. (2009). Supramarginal gyrus involvement in visual word recognition. *Cortex,* 45(9), 1091-1096.

Stoodley, C. J. (2012). The cerebellum and cognition: Evidence from functional imaging studies. *Cerebellum,* 11(2), 352–365.

Stoodley, C. J. and Schmahmann, J. D. (2009). Functional topography in the human cerebellum: A meta-analysis of neuroimaging studies. *NeuroImage,* 44, 489–501.

Stoodley, C. J., Valera, E. M. and Schmahmann, J. D. (2012). Functional topography of the cerebellum for motor and cognitive tasks: an fMRI study. *Neuroimage,* 59(2), 1560-1570.

Taipale, M., Kaminen, N., Nopola-Hemmi, J., Haltia, T., Myllyluoma, B., Lyytinen, H., Muller, K., Kaaranen, M., Lindsberg, P. J., Hannula-Jouppi, K., and Kere, J. (2003). A candidate gene for developmental dyslexia encodes a nuclear tetratricopeptide repeat domain protein dynamically regulated in brain. *Proceedings of the National Academy of Science of the US,* 100(20), 11553-11558.

Talairach, J. and Tournoux, P. (1988). *Co-planar stereotaxic atlas of the human brain.* New York: Thieme Medical Publishers.

Talcott, J. B., Witton, C., Hebb, G. S., Stoodley, C. J., Westwood, E. A., France, S. J., Hansen, P. C., and Stein, J. F. (2002). On the relationship between dynamic visual and auditory processing and literacy skills; results from a large primary-school study. *Dyslexia,* 8(4), 204-225.

Talcott, J. B., Witton, C., McLean, M. F., Hansen, P. C., Ress, A., Green, G. G. R., and Stein, J. F. (2000). Dynamic sensory sensitivity and children's word decoding skills. *Proceedings of the National Academy of Sciences (US),* 97, 2952–2957.

Temple, E. (2002). Brain mechanisms in normal and dyslexic readers. *Current Opinion in Neurobiology,* 12, 178-183.

Temple, E., Deutsch, G. K., Poldrack, R. A., Miller, S. L., Tallal, P., Merzenich, M. M., and Gabrieli, J. D. (2003). Neural deficits in children with dyslexia ameliorated by behavioral remediation: evidence from functional MRI. *Proc. Natl. Acad. Sci. US,* 100(5), 2860-2865.

Tessier-Lavigne, M. (2000). Visual processing by the retina. In: E. R. Kandel and J. H. Schwartz and T. M. Jessell (Eds.), *Principles of neural science* (pp. 507-522). New York: McGraw-Hill.

The FIL Methods Group. (2006). *SPM5 Manual.* London: Wellcome Department of Imaging Neuroscience Institute of Neurology, UCL.

Thomas, C. J. (1905). Congenital 'word-blindness' and its treatment. *Opthalmoscope,* 3, 380-385.

Tivarus, M. E., Hillier, A., Schmalbrock, P., and Beversdorf, D. Q. (2008). Functional connectivity in an fMRI study of semantic and phonological processes and the effect of L-Dopa. *Brain Lang.,* 104(1), 42-50.

Tootell, R. B., Mendola, J. D., Hadjikhani, N. K., Ledden, P. J., Liu, A. K., Reppas, J. B., Sereno, M. I., and Dale, A. M. (1997). Functional analysis of V3A and related areas in human visual cortex. *J. Neurosci.,* 17(18), 7060-7078.

Tootell, R. B. H. and Taylor, J. B. (1995). Anatomical evidence for MT and additional cortical visual areas in humans. *Cerebral Cortex,* 1, 39-55.

Torgesen, J. K., Wagner, R. K. and Rashotte, C. A. (1999). *Test of word reading efficiency.* Austin, Texas, US: Pro-ed.

Turkeltaub, P. E., Eden, G. F., Jones, K. M., and Zeffiro, T. A. (2002). Meta-analysis of the functional neuroanatomy of single-word reading: method and validation. *Neuroimage,* 16 (3 Pt 1), 765-780.

Tzourio-Mazoyer, N., Landeau, B., Papathanassiou, D., Crivello, F., Etard, O., Delcroix, N., Mazoyer, B., and Joliot, M. (2002). Automated anatomical labeling of activations in SPM using a macroscopic anatomical parcellation of the MNI MRI single-subject brain. *NeuroImage,* 15, 273–289.

Ugurbil, K. (2002). High-field magnetic resonance. In: A. W. Toga and J. C. Mazziotta (Eds.), *Brain mapping: The methods* (Second ed., pp. 291-313). San Diego, US: Academic Press.

Vandermosten, M., Boets, B., Poelmans, H., Sunaert, S., Wouters, J., and Ghesquiere, P. (2012). A tractography study in dyslexia: neuroanatomic correlates of orthographic, phonological and speech processing. *Brain,* 135(Pt 3), 935-948.

Vanni, S., Uusitalo, M. A., Kiesila, P., and Hari, R. (1997). Visual motion activates V5 in dyslexics. *Neuroreport,* 8(8), 1939-1942.

Vellutino, F. R. (1979). *Dyslexia: Research and theory.* Cambridge MA: MIT Press.

Vellutino, F. R., Fletcher, J. M., Snowling, M. J., and Scanlon, D. M. (2004). Specific reading disability (dyslexia): what have we learnt in the past four decades? *Journal of Child Psychology and Psychiatry,* 45, 2-40.

Venezky, R. L. (1970). *The structure of English orthography.* The Hague: Mouton.

Vinegrad, M. (1994). A revised Adult Dyslexia Check List. *Educare,* 48 21-23.

Wagner, R. K., Torgesen, J. K. and Rashotte, C. A. (1999). *CTOPP. Comprehensive test of phonological processing.* Austin, Texas, US: Pro-ED.

Wang, V. Y. and Zoghbi, H. Y. (2001). Genetic regulation of cerebellar development. *Nature Reviews Neuroscience,* 2(7), 484-491.

Wang, Y., Paramasivam, M., Thomas, A., Bai, J., Kaminen-Ahola, N., Kere, J., Voskuil, J., Rosen, G. D., Galaburda, A. M., and Loturco, J. J. (2006). DYX1C1 functions in neuronal migration in developing neocortex. *Neuroscience,* 143(2), 515-522.

Warrington, E. K., Logue, V. and Pratt, R. T. C. (1971). The anatomical localisation of selective impairment of auditory verbal short-term memory. *Neuropsychologia,* 9, 377-387.

Watson, J. D. G., Myers, R., Frackowiak, R. S. J., Hajnal, J. V., Woods, R. P., Mazziotta, J. C., Shipp, S., and Zeki, S. (1993). Area V5 of the human brain: Evidence from a combined study using positron emission tomography and magnetic resonance imaging. *Cerebral Cortex,* 3, 79-94.

Wechsler, D. (1997). *The Wechsler Adult Intelligence Scale - III*. London: The Psychological Corporation.

Wechsler, D. (1999). *The Wechsler Abbreviated Scale of Intelligence*. London: The Psychological Corporation.

White, S., Frith, U., Milne, E., Rosen, S., Swettenham, J., and Ramus, F. (2008). A double dissociation between sensorimotor impairments and reading disability: A comparison of autistic and dyslexic children. *Cognitive Neuropsychology,* 23(5), 748-761.

White, S., Milne, E., Rosen, S., Hansen, P., Swettenham, J., Frith, U., and Ramus, F. (2006). The role of sensorimotor impairments in dyslexia: A multiple case study of dyslexic children. *Developmental Science,* 9(3), 237–269.

Wilcke, A., Ligges, C., Burkhardt, J., Alexander, M., Wolf, C., Quente, E., Ahnert, P., Hoffmann, P., Becker, A., Muller-Myhsok, B., Cichon, S., Boltze, J., and Kirsten, H. (2012). Imaging genetics of FOXP2 in dyslexia. *Eur. J. Hum. Genet.,* 20(2), 224-229.

Wilkinson, G. S. (1993). *The Wide Range Achievement Test 3*. Wilmington, DE: Wide Range.

Willcutt, E. G. and Pennington, B. F. (2000). Comorbidity of reading disability and attention-deficit/hyperactivity disorder: Differences by gender and subtype. *Journal of Learning Disabilities* 33, 179-191.

Willcutt, E. G., Pennington, B. F. and DeFries, J. C. (2000). Twin study of the etiology of comorbidity between reading disability and attention-deficit/hyperactivity disorder. *Am. J. Med. Genet.,* 96(3), 293-301.

Willcutt, E. G., Pennington, B. F., Olson, R. K., Chhabildas, N., and Hulslander, J. (2005). Neuropsychological analyses of comorbidity between reading disability and attention deficit hyperactivity disorder: in search of the common deficit. *Dev. Neuropsychol.,* 27(1), 35-78.

Willcutt, E. G., Pennington, B. F., Smith, S. D., Cardon, L. R., Gayan, J., Knopik, V. S., Olson, R. K., and DeFries, J. C. (2002). Quantitative trait locus for reading disability on chromosome 6p is pleiotropic for attention-deficit/hyperactivity disorder. *Am. J. Med. Genet. (Neuropsychiatric Genetics),* 114(3), 260-268.

Wimmer, H., Mayringer, H. and Raberger, T. (1999). Reading and dual-task balancing: evidence against the automatization deficit explanation of developmental dyslexia. *J. Learn. Disabil.,* 32(5), 473-478.

Wolff, P. H., Cohen, C. and Drake, C. (1984). Impaired motor timing control in specific reading retardation. *Neuropsychologia,* 22(5), 587-600.

World Federation of Neurology. (1968). *Report of research group on dyslexia and world illiteracy*. Dallas: WFN.

Wurtz, R. H. and Kandel, E. R. (2000). Perception of motion, depth and form. In: E. R. Kandel and J. H. Schwartz and T. M. Jessell (Eds.), *Principles of neural science* (4th ed., pp. 548-571). New York: McGraw-Hill.

Xu, B., Grafman, J., Gaillard, W. D., Ishii, K., Vega-Bermudez, F., Pietrini, P., Reeves-Tyler, P., DiCamillo, P., and Theodore, W. (2001). Conjoint and extended neural networks for the computation of speech codes: The neural basis of selective impairment in reading words and pseudowords. *Cerebral Cortex,* 11, 267-277.

Zatorre, R. J. and Gandour, J. T. (2009). Neural specializations for speech and pitch: Moving beyond the dichotomies. In: B. C. Moore and L. K. Tyler and W. D. Marslen-Wilson (Eds.), *The perception of speech* (pp. 275-304). Oxford: Oxford University Press.

Zeki, S., Watson, J. D., Lueck, C. J., Friston, K. J., Kennard, C., and Frackowiak, R. S. (1991). A direct demonstration of functional specialization in human visual cortex. *J. Neurosci.,* 11(3), 641-649.

Zheng, N. and Raman, I. M. (2010). Synaptic inhibition, excitation, and plasticity in neurons of the cerebellar nuclei. *Cerebellum,* 9(1), 56-66.

Zhu, Y., Li, H., Zhou, L., Wu, J. Y., and Rao, Y. (1999). Cellular and molecular guidance of GABAergic neuronal migration from an extracortical origin to the neocortex. *Neuron,* 23, 473-485.

Zilles, K., Schleicher, A., Palomero-Gallagher, N., and Amunts, K. (2002). Quantitative analysis of cyto- and receptor architecture of the human brain. In: J. Mazziotta and A. Toga (Eds.), *Brain Mapping. The Methods* (2nd ed., pp. 573 - 602): Elsevier.

In: Advances in Neuroimaging Research
Editor: Victoria Asher-Hansley

ISBN: 978-1-63321-307-4

Chapter II

QEEG/LORETA Electrical Imaging in Neuropsychiatry-Diagnosis and Treatment Implications

J. Lucas Koberda*, M.D., Ph.D.
Professor of Neurology and Director of
Tallahassee NeuroBalance Center, Tallahassee, FL, US
www.TallahasseeNeuroBalanceCenter.com

Abstract

Quantitative Electroencephalography (QEEG) combined with Low Resolution Electro-magnetic Tomography Analysis (QEEG/LORETA) is a relatively new form of functional imaging which is able to indicate which region of the brain is malfunctioning and contributing to a patient's symptoms. In contrast to functional MRI, PET and SPECT imaging, which measure secondary metabolic processes, QEEG/LORETA records direct neuronal activity through the surface of the head. Introduction of QEEG/LORETA brain imaging has improved our diagnostic ability in neuropsychiatric practice by identifying dysregulated cortical areas implicated in patient's symptoms. Additional use of LORETA Z-score neurofeedback (NFB) enables us to directly target these areas of dysregulation in order to improve associated symptoms. Based on approximately 250 patients treated in our clinic with Z-score LORETA NFB, a detailed analysis of selected cases is presented. Cases include depression/anxiety, chronic pain, epilepsy, ADHD and cognitive dysfunction. Specific areas of dysregulation attributed to particular conditions identified by LORETA are presented: Anterior Cingulate and Insular cortex in pain syndromes; as well as specific Brodmann's Areas in other cases. Follow up findings of QEEG/LORETA electrical imaging after NFB and computerized cognitive testing are discussed. In addition, cases of Z-score LORETA NFB mediated cognitive enhancement are shown. This chapter encompasses examples of the application of functional neurology in neuropsychiatry.

* Phone-(850) 877-2802; Fax-(850) 222-1383. Email: JLKoberda@yahoo.com.

Keywords: EEG, QEEG, LORETA, Electrical Imaging, Neuropsychiatry, Neurofeedback

Introduction

German physiologist and psychiatrist Hans Berger (1873–1941) recorded the first human EEG in 1924 (Haas, L F, 2003). Expanding on work previously conducted on animals by Richard Caton and others, Dr. Berger also invented the electroencephalogram (giving the device its name), an invention described "as one of the most surprising, remarkable, and momentous developments in the history of clinical neurology" (Haas, L F, 2003).

Electroencephalography (EEG) is the recording of electrical activity along the scalp. The meninges, cerebrospinal fluid and skull "smear" the EEG signal, obscuring its intracranial source. In clinical contexts, EEG refers to the recording of the brain's spontaneous electrical activity over a short period of time, usually 20–40 minutes, as recorded from multiple electrodes placed on the scalp (Niedermeyer E. and da Silva F.L., 2004).

The electric potential generated by an individual neuron is far too small to be picked up by EEG (Nunez PL, Srinivasan R, 1981). EEG activity therefore always reflects the summation of the synchronous activity of thousands or millions of neurons that have similar spatial orientation.

EEG is most often used to diagnose epilepsy, which causes obvious abnormalities in EEG readings (Niedermeyer E. and da Silva F.L. 2004). It is also used to diagnose sleep disorders, coma, encephalopathies, and brain death. EEGs were formally first-line method of diagnosis for tumors, stroke and other focal brain disorders (Niedermeyer E. and da Silva F.L. 2004); this use has decreased with the advent of high-resolution anatomical imaging techniques such as MRI and CT. Despite limited spatial resolution, EEG continues to be a valuable tool for research and diagnosis, especially when millisecond-range temporal resolution (not possible with CT or MRI) is required.

Computed tomography (CT) and magnetic resonance imaging (MRI) may be viewed as imaging type which can reveal mostly structure of the brain. Intermediate time-scale methods like functional magnetic resonance imaging (fMRI) and positron emission tomography (PET) track brain changes over seconds or minutes, while supplying more information on the function of the brain. EEG and QEEG provide more functional information on much faster time scales in milliseconds (Nunez, P.L. et al. 2014). Quantitative electroencephalography (QEEG) is a non-invasive technique that allows a highly precise measurement of brain function and connectivity (Billeci L, et al. 2013). QEEG is defined as the mathematical processing of digitally recorded EEG in order to highlight specific waveform components, transform the EEG into a format or domain that elucidates relevant information, or associate numerical results (Nuwer M, 2007). Therefore, QEEG applies computerized mathematical algorithms to transform raw EEG data into a number of frequency bands of interest (Billeci L, et al. 2013). Five wide frequency bands are usually studied, typically defined as delta (1–4 Hz), theta (4–8 Hz), alpha (8–12 Hz), beta (12–30 Hz), and gamma (over 30 Hz). The same defined frequency bands will be used in the rest of this chapter. Usefulness of QEEG in neurological diagnosis and treatment was addressed and confirmed in one of my prior papers (Koberda et al. 2013).

Low Resolution Electromagnetic Tomography Analysis (LORETA) Imaging

To localize the cortical sources of scalp EEG activity we used low resolution electromagnetic tomography analysis (Pascual-Marqui RD et al. 1994). The low resolution electromagnetic tomography analysis (LORETA) method is a discrete, three-dimensional (3D) distributed, linear, inverse solution. The smoothing constraints in LORETA endows the tomography with the property of low localization errors to test point sources, albeit with low spatial resolution (i.e. neighbouring neuronal sources will be highly correlated (Pascual-Marqui RD et al. 1994). The LORETA inverse solution corresponds to the 3D distribution of electrical neuronal activity that features a maximum similarity (i.e. maximum synchronization), in term of orientation and strength, between neuronal populations in adjacent voxels. The imaging is therefore particularly tuned towards synchronized brain activities as they occur, e.g. in spreading oscillatory activations. Since LORETA takes explicitly into account that scalp electric potentials are determined up to an arbitrary additive constant, the final LORETA solution is independent of the electrical reference used. Deep structures such as the anterior cingulate cortex (Pizzagalli D, et al. 2001) insula and mesial temporal lobes (Zumsteg D et al. 2006) can be correctly localized with LORETA.

The following case will demonstrate superiority of QEEG/LORETA electrical imaging over "structural" MRI brain imaging in detection of brain dysfunction.

Case 1

Fifty four year old male with college education was seen in my office and reporting four years history of gradual decline of his cognitive function including short-term memory. His cognitive problems resulted in his job termination two years ago. His MRI of the brain was reported as normal by neuro-radiologist (see Figure 1).

Subsequent computerized cognitive testing (Neurotrax, Inc) showed evidence of low cognitive score: Global Cognitive Score (GCS)-65.6, memory-54.3, executive function-62.4, Attention-42.8, Information Processing Speed-70.5, Visual Spatial-104.1, Verbal Function-59.4. (Expected score mean-100 with standard deviation-15). QEEG and LORETA functional analysis revealed evidence of mostly increased frontal beta power with milder increase in frontal delta and theta power (Figure 2). LORETA showed several areas of electrical dysregulation including frontal and temporal lobes with Brodmann's areas 8, 9 and 38 (Figure 3). Abnormalities in amplitude asymmetry, coherence and phase lag were also noted. Dysregulations of BA 8, 9 and 38 may be seen in patients with cognitive and memory problems (Kübler A et al, 2006, Zhang JX, et al. 2003, Brunet E, et al. 2000). There was marked hypo- and hyper-coherence, suggesting dysfunctional inter-hemispheric connectivity between neurons. Phase lag measurements were also abnormal, and this reflects conduction problems between two points that are engaged in similar brain activity. Grossly abnormal QEEG and LORETA testing validates that there is a visible close corelation between patient symptoms, cognitive testing and electrical imaging. This case is an example emphasizing importance of choosing appropriate test in order to confirm cognitive dysfunction and visualize functional abnormlities existing despite normal structural imaging.

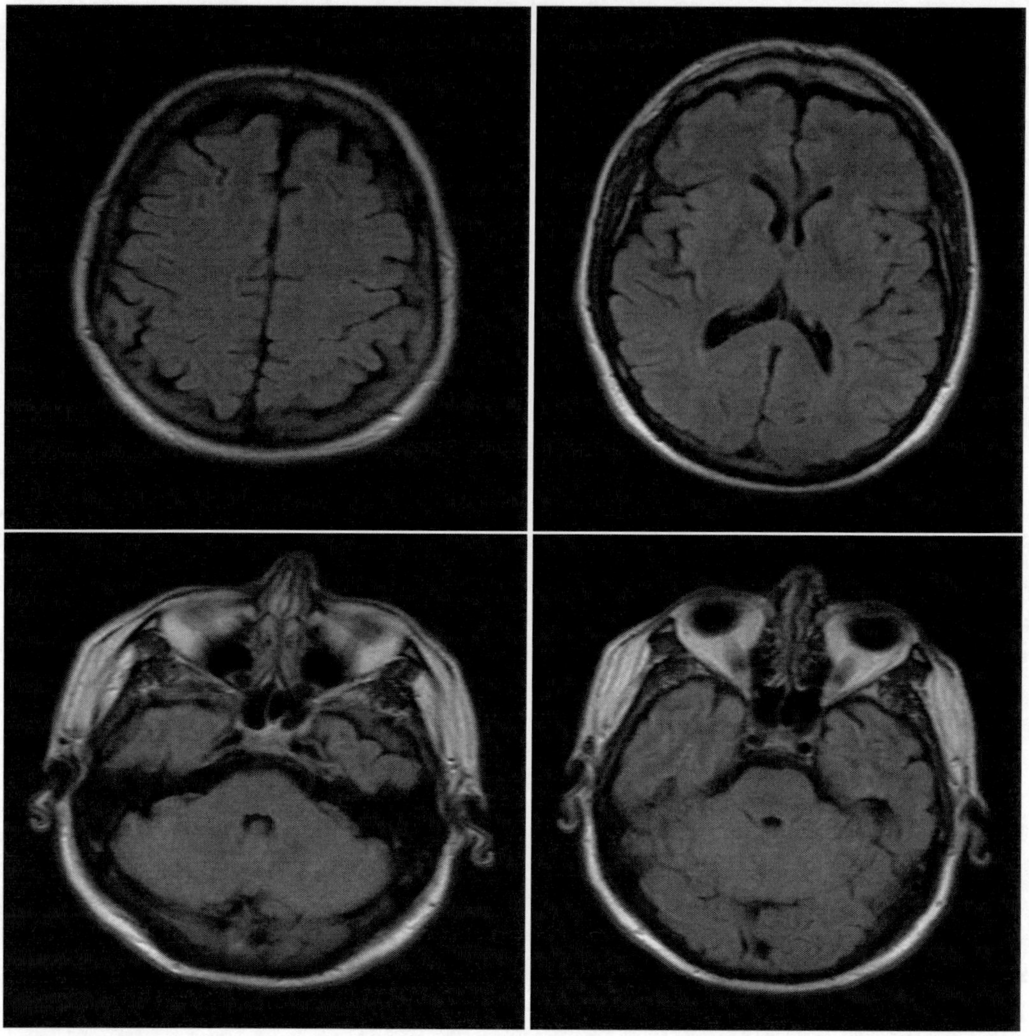

Figure 1. MRI of 54 year old male (4 different slices) with 4 years history of gradual cognitive decline (reported as normal).

Z-score LORETA Imaging and Biofeedback

EEG biofeedback (NFB), also called neurofeedback, is a type of biofeedback that uses real-time displays of EEG to illustrate brain activity and teach self-regulation.

EEG biofeedback has resulted in a wide range of biofeedback approaches, but many good clinical outcomes required more than 50 to 80 sessions.

However, the goal is to achieve good clinical outcome in fewer sessions. Real-time fMRI biofeedback can achieve modification of blood flow and regulate the activity in specific brain regions, e.g., amygdala in patients with depression (Young KD et al. 2014). Despite the fact that fMRI signal-Blood Oxygen Level Dependent (BOLD) is an indirect measure, there is growing evidence for a strong correlation between the BOLD signal and electrical brain activity (Sitaram R et al. 2007).

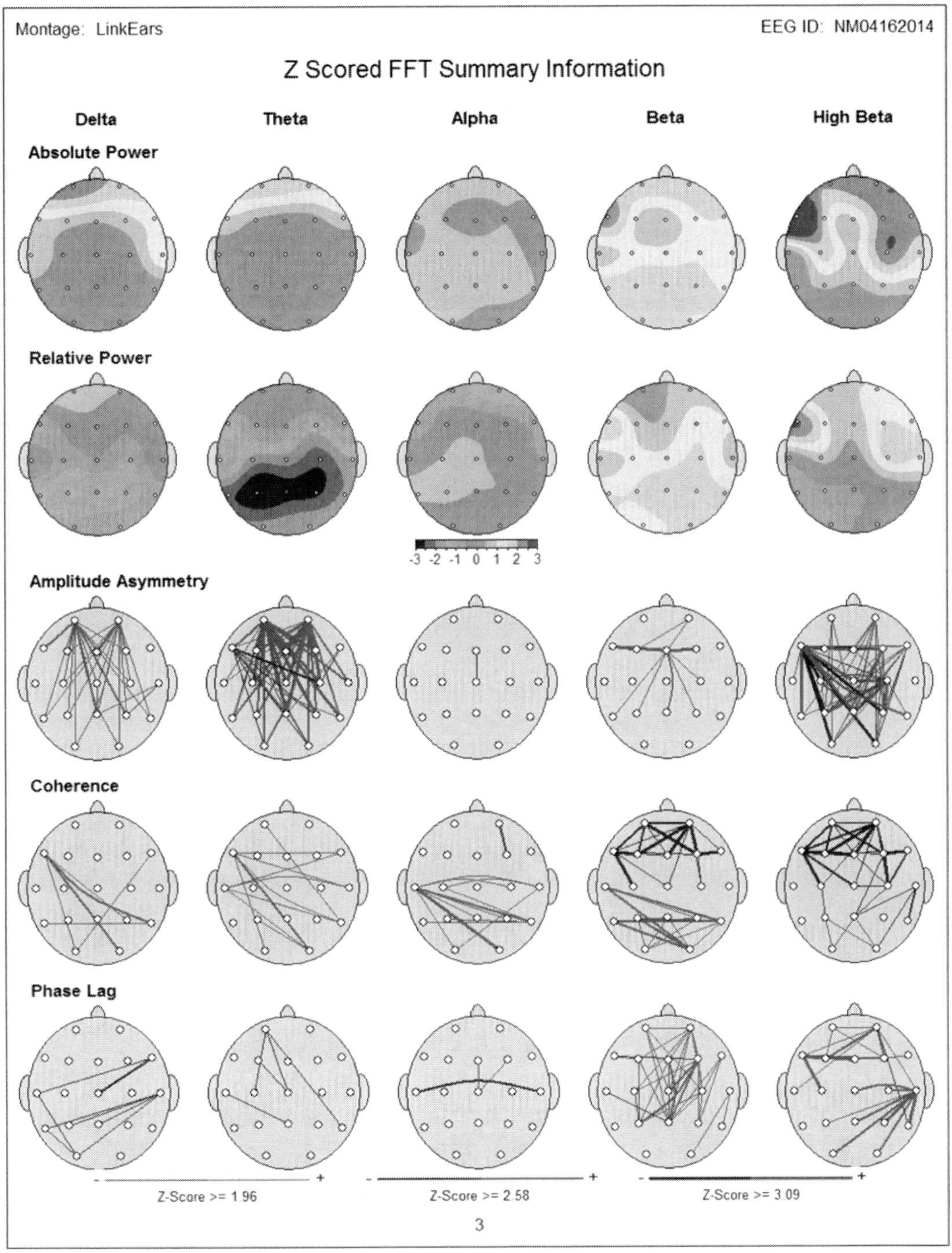

Figure 2. QEEG of 54 year old male with 4 years history of gradual cognitive decline. Marked increase in frontal beta, delta and theta power is noted (depicted in red or darker color for B/W images).

Studies have characterized the relationship between localized increases in neuronal activity and the corresponding increase in BOLD (Logothetis et al. 2001], Shmuel et al. 2006), making it possible to interpret positive functional responses in terms of neural changes. However, high costs associated with fMRI use are considered as one of prohibitive causes limiting its use in clinical settings. Therefore, LORETA EEG-biofeedback, which can be applied with relatively low cost at any clinic, seems to be superior for accomplishing a self-regulation of the brain.

In the 1990s, a new form of EEG biofeedback (Z-score biofeedback) was suggested, in which real-time comparisons to an age matched reference population of healthy or normal subjects are used as a guide or "compass" to increase specificity and provide a uniform direction and threshold for the biofeedback process (Thatcher, 2012). Prior to Z score biofeedback clinicians had to guess about what threshold to set for a given frequency or location to trigger the feedback signal or reinforcer signal (Thatcher, 2012).

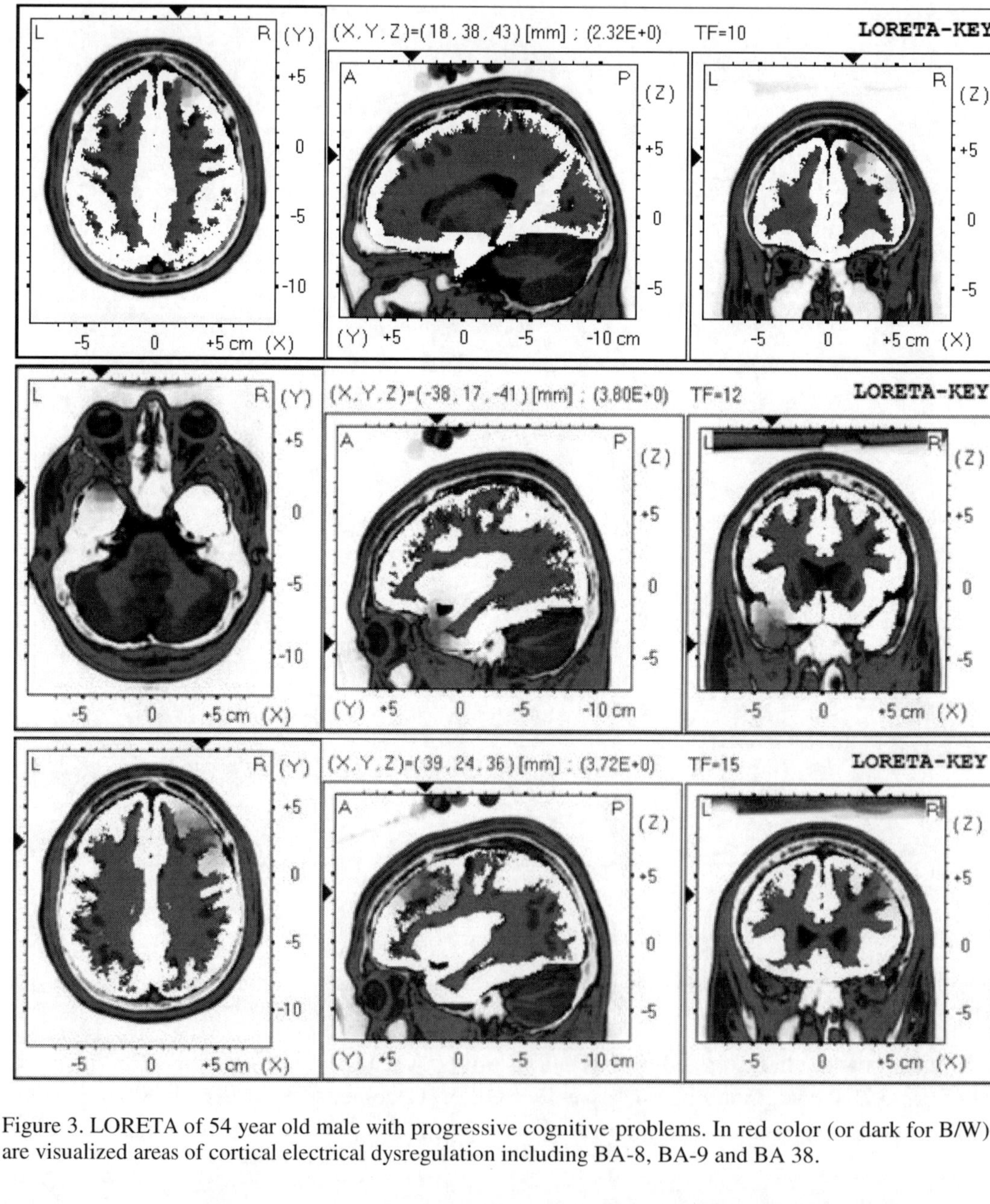

Figure 3. LORETA of 54 year old male with progressive cognitive problems. In red color (or dark for B/W) are visualized areas of cortical electrical dysregulation including BA-8, BA-9 and BA 38.

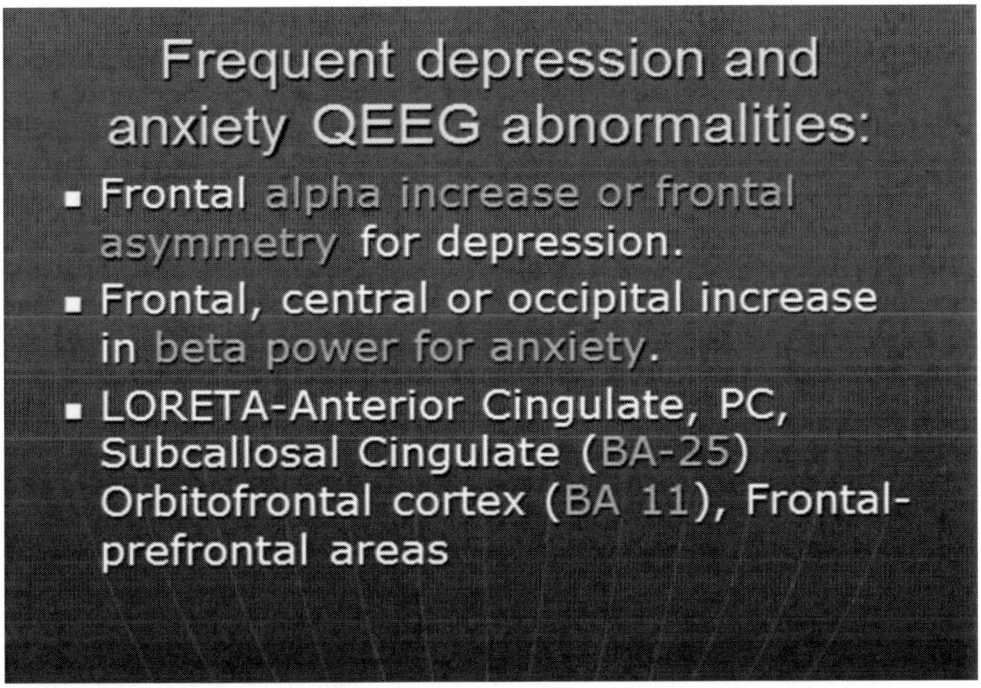

Figure 4 A. Summary of frequently identified QEEG/LORETA abnormalities in patients suffering from depression and anxiety:

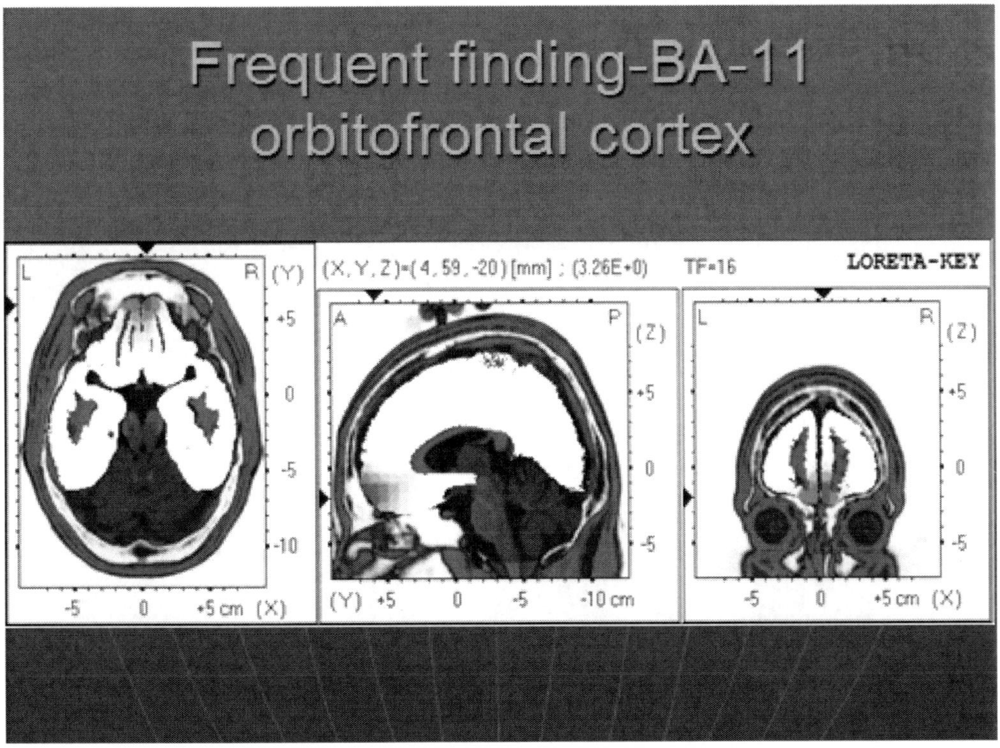

Figure 4 B. Orbitofrontal electrical (area in red) dysregulation (BA-11) seen in one of the patients with depression and anxiety.

Z score biofeedback greatly simplifies and standardizes EEG biofeedback by reducing many different metrics (absolute power, relative power, ratios, coherence, phase) to a single or common metric of the Z score or a standard deviation with respect to the EEG from a group of age matched healthy normal subjects (Thatcher, 2012).

Surface Z scores improve specificity by isolating dysregulated locations and rhythms, especially when using the Laplacian transform and LORETA Z scores are even more specific. For example, LORETA Z score biofeedback often also produces results in one 20 minute session because EEG source localization has accuracies of about 1 cm to 3 cm and thus is much more specific than is surface EEG (Thatcher RW, 2012).

In Z-Score NFB, a real-time comparison to an age-matched population of healthy subjects is used for data acquisition, simplifying protocol generation and allowing clinicians to target modules and hubs that indicate dysregulation and instability in networks related to symptoms (Thatcher, 2013). Z-score NFB increases specificity in operant conditioning, providing a guide that links extreme Z-score outliers to symptoms, and then reinforcing Z-score shifts toward states of greater homeostasis and stability. The goal is increased efficiency of information processing in brain networks related to the patient's symptoms (Thatcher, 2013).

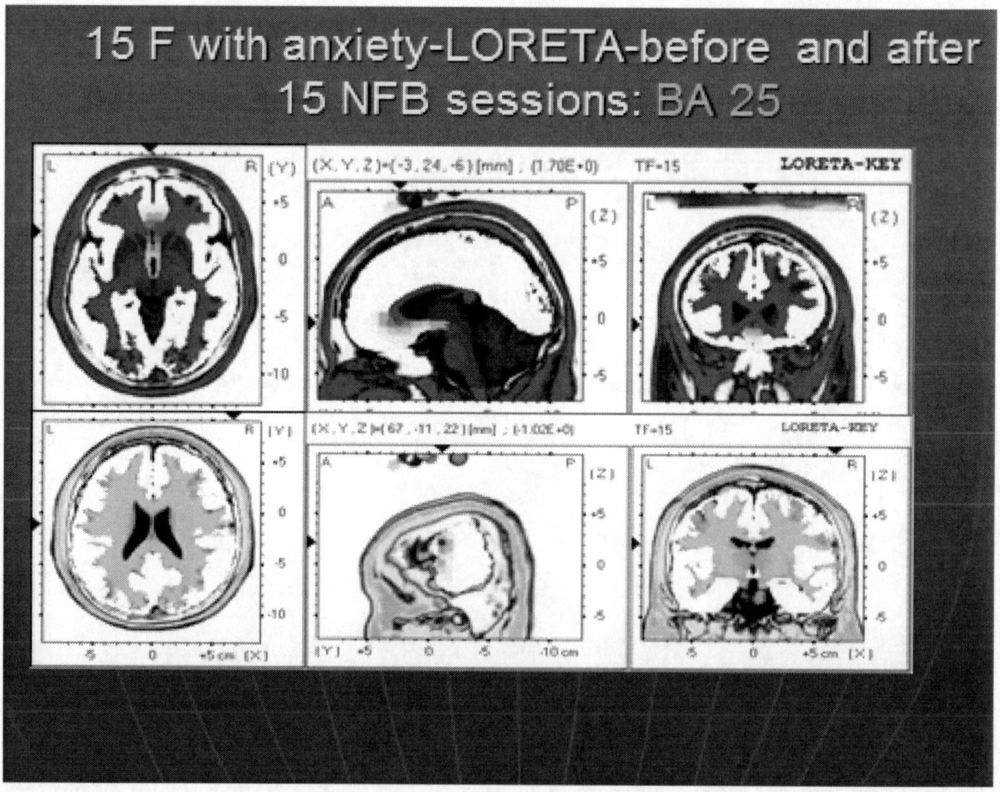

Figure 5 B. (Continued).

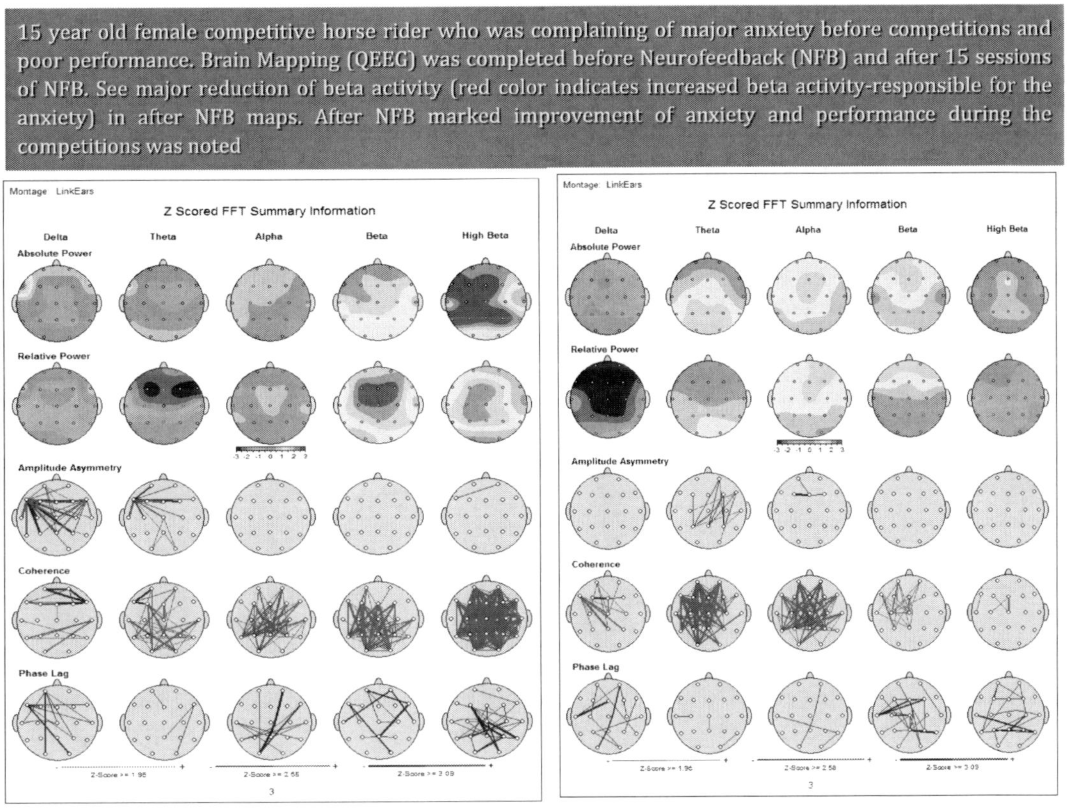

Figure 5 B. QEEG maps of 15 Y.O. female suffering from anxiety. Left image shows brain maps before NFB, right image shows brain maps after 15 NFB sessions.

A recently introduced method called Low Resolution Electromagnetic Tomography (LORETA) Z-score NFB is capable of targeting specific dysregulated anatomical structures, many of which are in deep cortical locations (Koberda et al., 2013; Thatcher, 2013). For example, the insula and anterior cingulate have been identified as potential NFB target sites for improving pain control in patients who display electrical dysregulation of these areas (Koberda et al. 2013).

My neurology center conducted Z-score LORETA NFB therapy for 31 patients with depression and/or associated anxiety. In addition to depression and anxiety, these patients frequently reported other coexisting problems including cognitive dysfunction, OCD and chronic pain (Koberda et al. 2014). Most patients were found to have QEEG abnormalities including alpha power increase, asymmetry, or LORETA electrical dysregulation in frontal areas (Figure 4 A and B).

Detailed analysis of my patients diagnosed with depression and/or anxiety showed that out of 31 included in the study, 24 (77%) were found to have both subjective and objective (improvement of QEEG abnormalities) improvement of the symptoms within 10 sessions of LORETA Z-score NFB (Koberda et al. 2014). In the next part of this chapter, I would like to present several cases selected from my practice illustrating application of LORETA imaging for diagnosis and subsequent NFB therapy.

Case 2

Figures 5 A and B show LORETA images, as well as brain maps, before and after completion of 15 sessions of Z-score LORETA NFB for a 15 year old female who suffered from extreme anxiety before and during horse riding competitions. Her symptoms included anxiety with palpitations, frequently associated with nausea and vomiting. Marked dysregulation of the anterior cingulate subcallosal region - Brodmann's Area (BA) 25 - was identified during the pre-NFB LORETA (Figure 5 A), manifesting as increased beta activity. Following 15 NFB sessions, this electrical dysregulation was corrected, as seen on the lower portion of the Figure 5 A. This was associated with diminishment of her symptoms and an improved performance in horse riding competitions.

Case 3

This is a 46-year-old female with 18 months history of the right trigeminal neuralgia. Patient has been taking pregabalin (Lyrica) 100 mg PO BID for neuralgic pain and duloxetine (Cymbalta) for depression and pain. Patient reported that despite taking increasing dose of Lyrica (previously was on 50 mg BID), the pain was not improving and she gained a lot of weight (her weight exceeded over 300 lb). Patient was interested in trying an alternative modality of therapy, exhibiting interest with starting Z-score LORETA NFB. Her initial QEEG showed elevation of frontal-temporal delta and theta power, as well as frontal beta power.

In addition, LORETA analysis showed an area of dysregulation in the left insular cortex (Figure 6). She reported marked pain improvement after the first session of NFB, and was able to reduce the dose of LYRICA after the second session and discontinue Lyrica completely after the 4th session. Patient completed 10 Sessions of NFB and has been in remission for over 4 months period. QEEG completed after total pain resolution showed an improvement in frontal delta, theta, and beta power, as well as a resolution of insular cortex dysregulation (Figure 7).

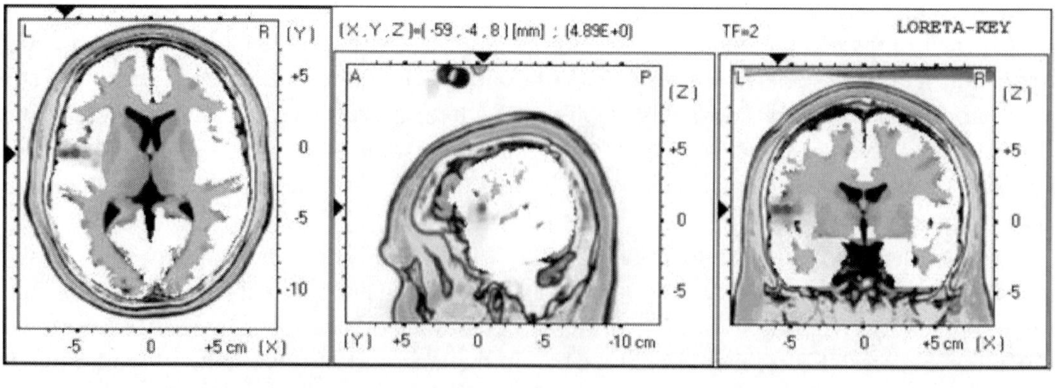

Figure 6. Before initiation of NFB LORETA showed area of dysregulation of the left insular cortex (in red).

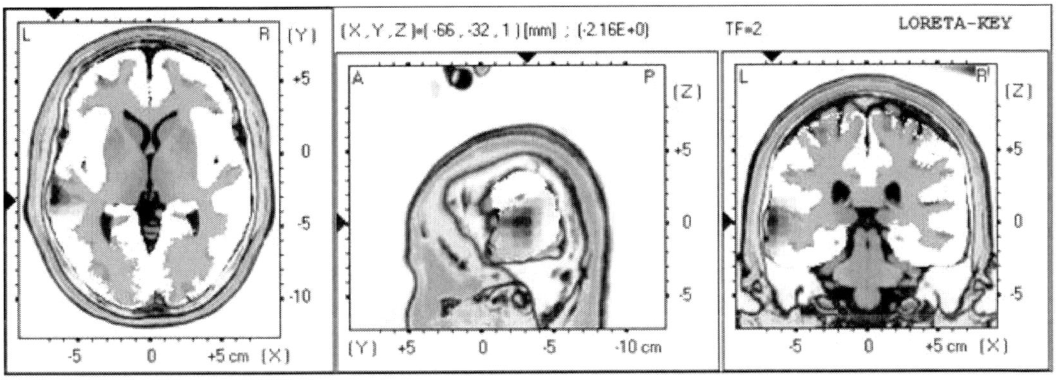

Figure 7. After NFB initiation and resolution of the pain LORETA showed no more evidence of the left insular cortex dysregulation.

Case 4

This is 65 year old male with long standing history of migraines and tension headaches frontal in location and sometimes lasting all day. Patient expressed interest in NFB since he noticed recent headaches exacerbation with poor response to medications. His QEEG showed increased frontal and central beta power and LORETA imaging indicated cingulate gyrus (BA-24) electrical dysregulation (Figure 8 A and B). Initial improvement of his headaches was noted after the first NFB session. After 10 sessions of LORETA Z-score NFB, his headaches markedly improved as well as frontal beta power (Figure 9). LORETA imaging after the course of NFB also showed resolution of previously dysregulated cortical electrical activity. Since this patient recently completed his therapy we are not sure how long will be his remission before possible headaches reoccurrence.

Case 5

An eight year old male with Attention Deficit Hyperactivity Disorder (ADHD) came with his mother for an examination. She described his problems at school, including learning and behavioral difficulties. He had trouble paying attention (resulting in poor grades), and was enrolled in the special education program at school. He had a history of speech delay, clumsiness, and was often fidgety and unable to sit still. The mother reported neither prior medical problems nor pregnancy complications. During the examination, he often interrupted and squirmed around in his chair; he was alert and able to follow instructions.

Before NFB therapy was initiated, the eight-year-old boy was tested using computerized neurocognitive testing. NeuroTrax is a computerized testing of cognitive functions, including memory, executive functioning, attention, information processing speed, visual spatial, verbal functioning, and motor skills. The test is scored based on the comparison to age and education matched controls with expected score of 100 and a standard deviation of 15. During the patient's first testing session before NFB, he scored 72.4 points overall (Global Cognitive Score), reflecting a below average score in every area except for verbal functioning (Table 1).

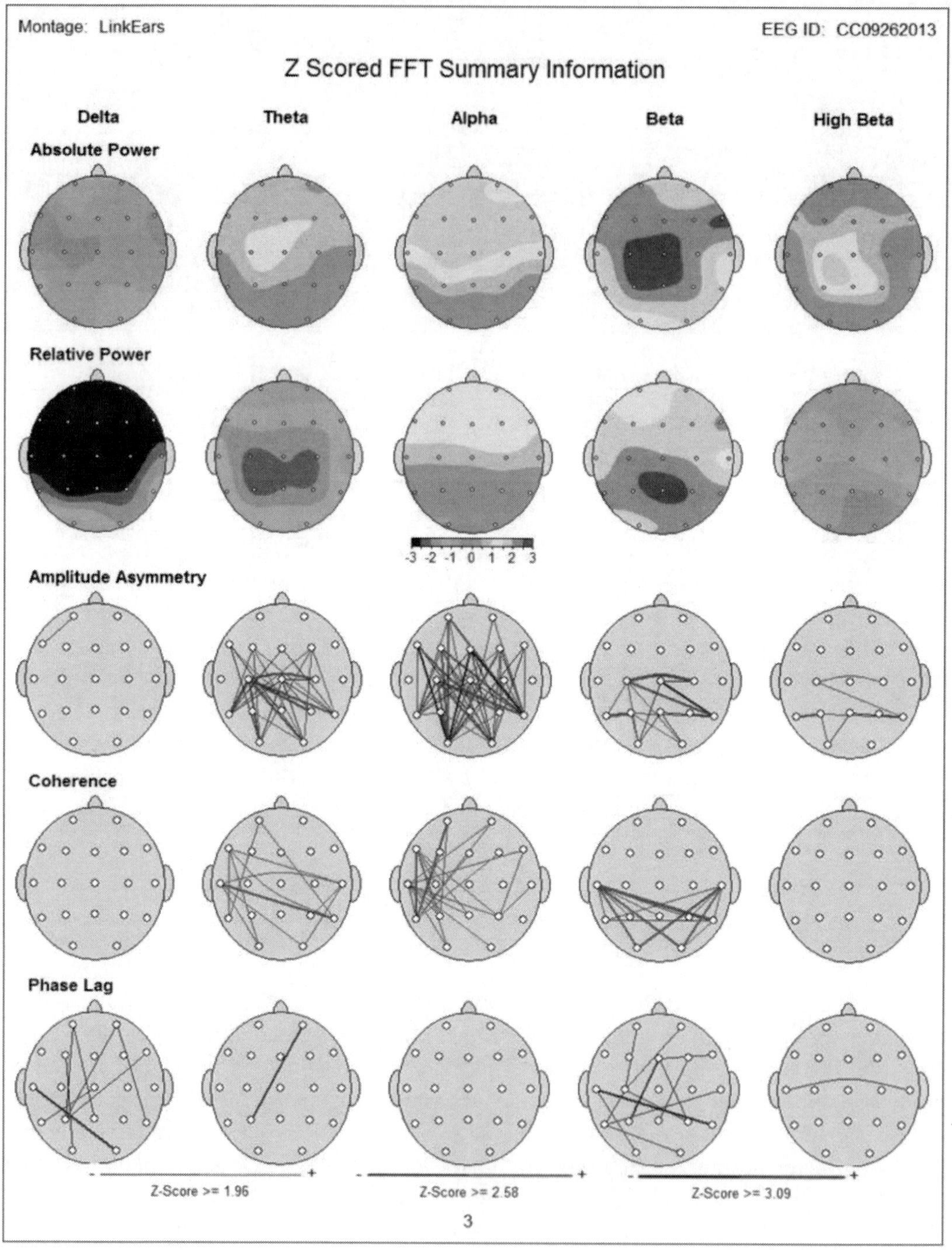
Montage: LinkEars
EEG ID: CC09262013
Z Scored FFT Summary Information
Delta
Theta
Alpha
Beta
High Beta
Absolute Power
Relative Power
-3 -2 -1 0 1 2 3
Amplitude Asymmetry
Coherence
Phase Lag
Z-Score >= 1.96
Z-Score >= 2.58
Z-Score >= 3.09
3

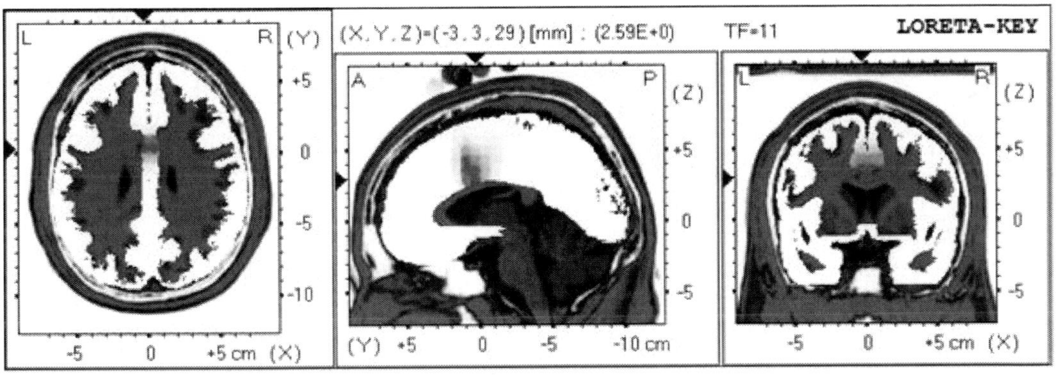

Figure 8. B-65 male with -before NFB-LORETA showed area of cortical dysfegulation in the cingulate region-BA-24 (in red) in alpha and beta frequency.

Table 1. Computerized neurocognitive testing (NeuroTrax) results before and after NFB initiation

Time	Jan 2013	March	June	Nov 2013
	0	12	30	60 NFB sessions
Global Cognitive Score	**72.4**	**80.1**	**85**	**94.1**
Memory	58.1	76.7	69.7	85.1
Executive Function	49.1	74	70.8	91.2
Attention	31.6	62.7	73.5	86
Info Processing Speed	-	-	-	73.9
Visual Spatial	97.7	92.7	97.7	118.6
Verbal Function	116.3	83.9	105.5	108.6
Motor Skills	81.3	90.4	92.5	95.5

Each time the patient came with his mother for NFB, they were first asked if any progress has been made in his behavior/school performance; their response was recorded as a subjective response.

After only 12 sessions of NFB, his NeuroTrax global cognitive score (GCS) rose to 80.1 points overall (Table 1). His memory score increased from 58.1 to 76.7, executive functioning from 49.1 to 74, and attention from 31.6 to 62.7. His family could see improvements with his vocabulary and overall functioning. He was tested again after another 18 sessions (total 30 sessions) scoring 85 points (GCS) on Neurotrax, and then another time after an additional 30 sessions (Table 1). After 60 NFB sessions, his GCS rose to 94.1 points on neurocognitive testing (Table 1). The patient's memory score was now 85.1, his executive functioning had reached 91.2 points, and his attention scored 86. His information processing speed (previously too low to score) now achieved 73.9 points, and his visual spatial score was above average at 118.6 points. In addition to marked improvement on the neurocognitive testing, academic performance in school grads also accelerated.

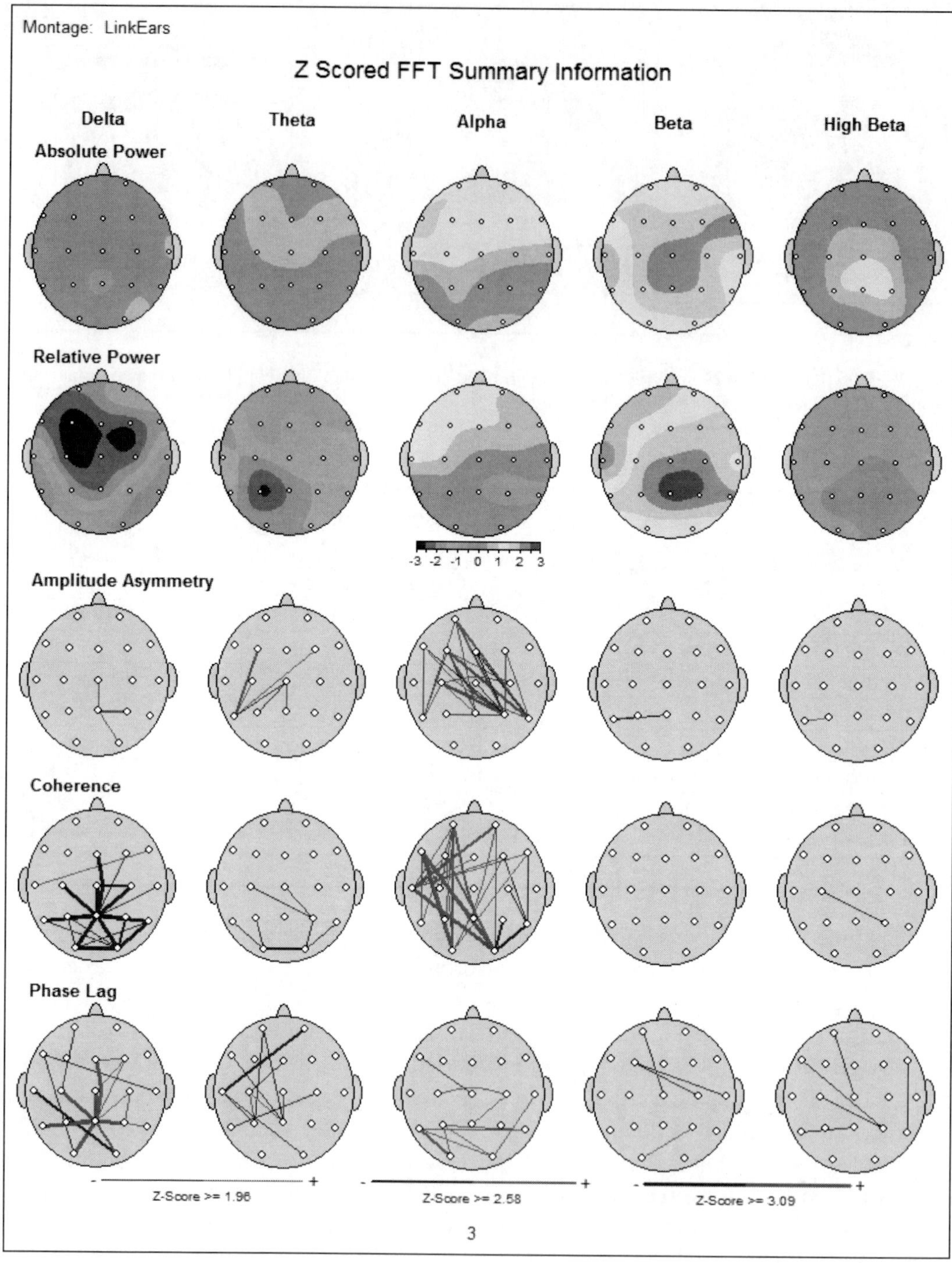

Figure 9. 65 year old with -after NFB-QEEG shows an improvement of previously overexpressed frontal and central beta power.

QEEG testing before Z-score LORETA NFB showed marked increase in frontal and central beta power (Figure 10 B). LORETA revealed an area of electrical dysregulation in the anteriot cingulate (AC) gyrus (Figure 10 A). Subsequent NFB sessions led to gradual improvement of the patient's school performance. After 10 sessions of therapy, QEEG findings indicated marked improvement of excessive beta activity (Figure 11). Further NFB therapy accomplished even better reduction of beta activity (Figure 12), and reduction of AC electrical dysregulation. However, some intermittent intersession fluctuation of beta power was also visible during the course of the treatment.

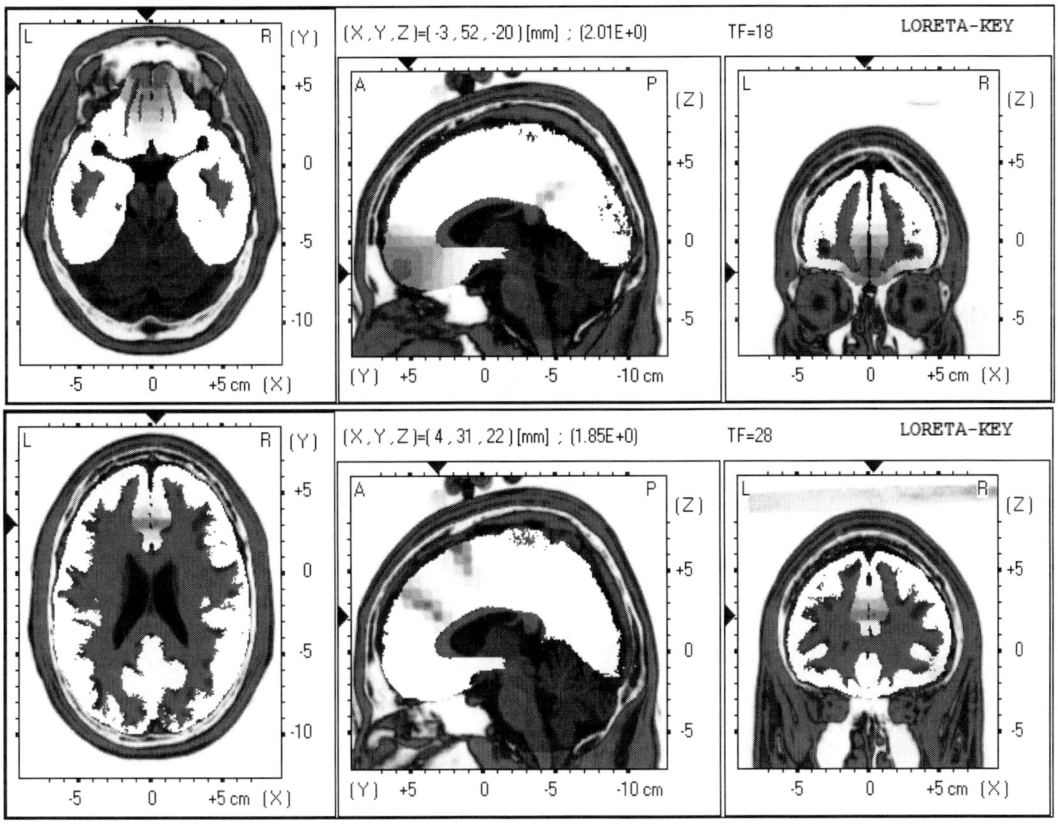

Figure 10 A. Before NFB-LORETA showed electrical dysregulation of anterior cingulate gyrus-(Brodmann's Area 32 and 24-seen in red) in beta frequency.

Figure 10. (Continued).

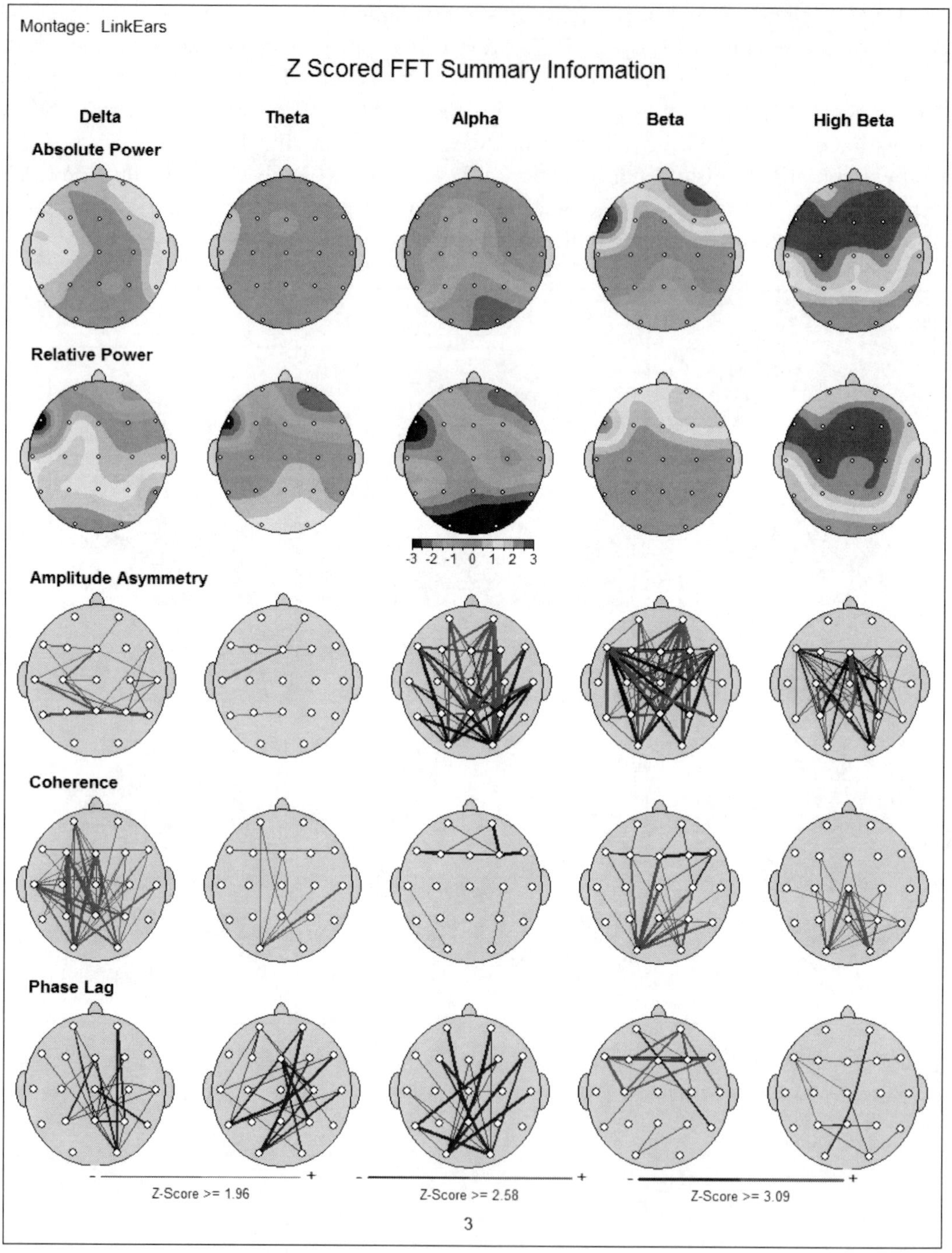

Figure 10 B. QEEG before NFB initiation. Noticeable prominent excess of frontal beta and high beta activity depicted in red color. Green color shows brain power within 1 standard deviation, yellow color within 2 standard deviations.

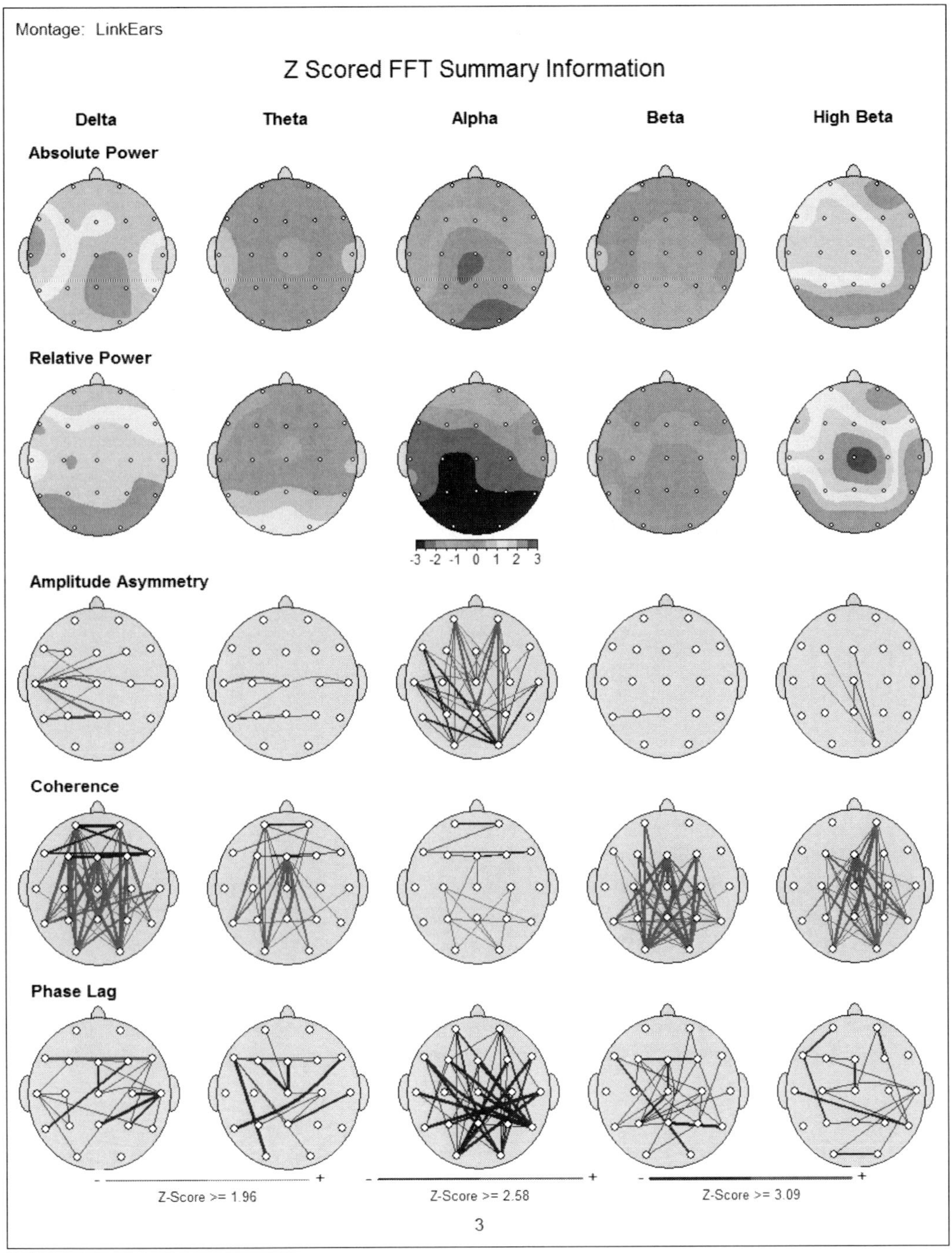

Figure 11. QEEG after 10 NFB sessions. Marked reduction of frontal beta and high beta power was recorded (reduction of red color or reduction of dark grey in B/W).

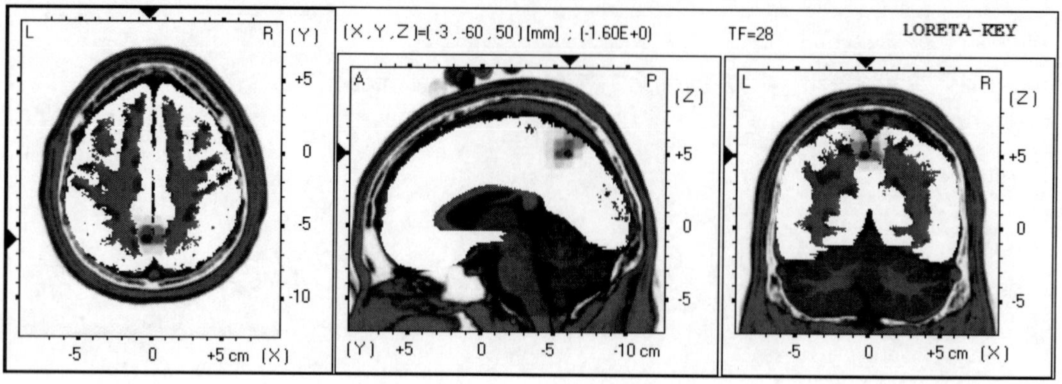

Figure 12. After 30 sessions of NFB LORETA shows no evidence any longer of anterior cingulate electrical dysregulation.

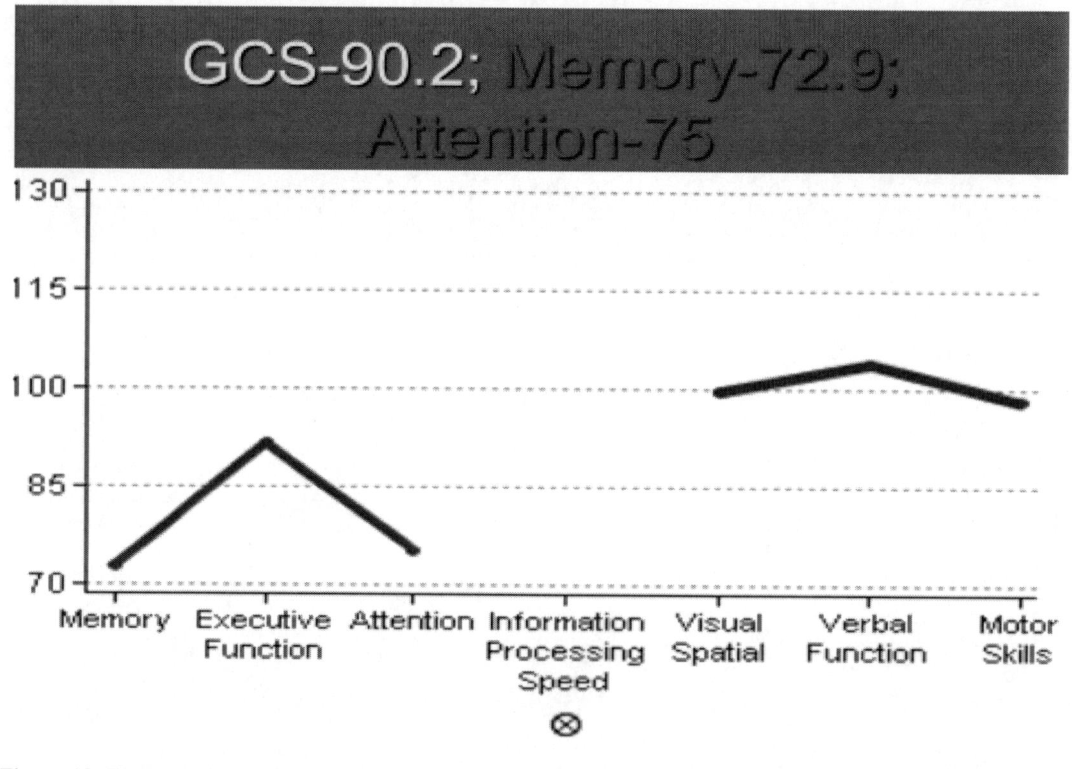

Figure 13. Illustrates lower than expected cognitive score especially memory and attention as well as information processing speed (too low to be scored). Expected score-100 with Standard Deviation (SD) -15. GCS-Global Cognitive Score.

Case 6

This is 18 year old female high school senior who's seizures started at age 11, sometimes proceeded by eye blinking episodes. Her current medications included Keppra XR 1500 mg daily and Lamictal 150 mg daily. Prior MRI-of the brain was reported to be normal. EEG showed multiple sharps in several locations including P3, P4 T5, T6, O1, O2. Cognitive testing showed low information processing speed and memory (Figure 13). Despite extensive neurological evaluations at UCLA and multiple medications initiation, no seizure reduction was observed. Her mother even reported an increase in seizure numbers with use of anti-epileptic mediations. Dr. Barry Sterman was also consulted and sensory-motor rhythm NFB was initiated with some seizure reduction noted. However, despite 90-100 sessions of NFB completion epilepsy fits were still occurring, but with lower frequency. This patient presented to my office for one week of intensive therapy with Z-score LORETA NFB (twice a day). LORETA imaging showed multiple areas of cortical electrical dysregulations (Figure 14). After completion of 8 NFB sessions longer remission was achieved (approximately 4 months). Further NFB therapy was however continued at another location but with much lower frequency. Since the initiation of Z-score LORETA NFB therapy (approximately 11 months) only 2 seizures were noted. In addition, marked improvement of cognitive status was found with resultant admission to college and very good grades during the freshmen year (mostly A's).

Case 7

Forty-year-old female, who was previously treated by psychiatrist for major depression and did not respond to pharmacological treatment, was referred to me for NFB treatment.

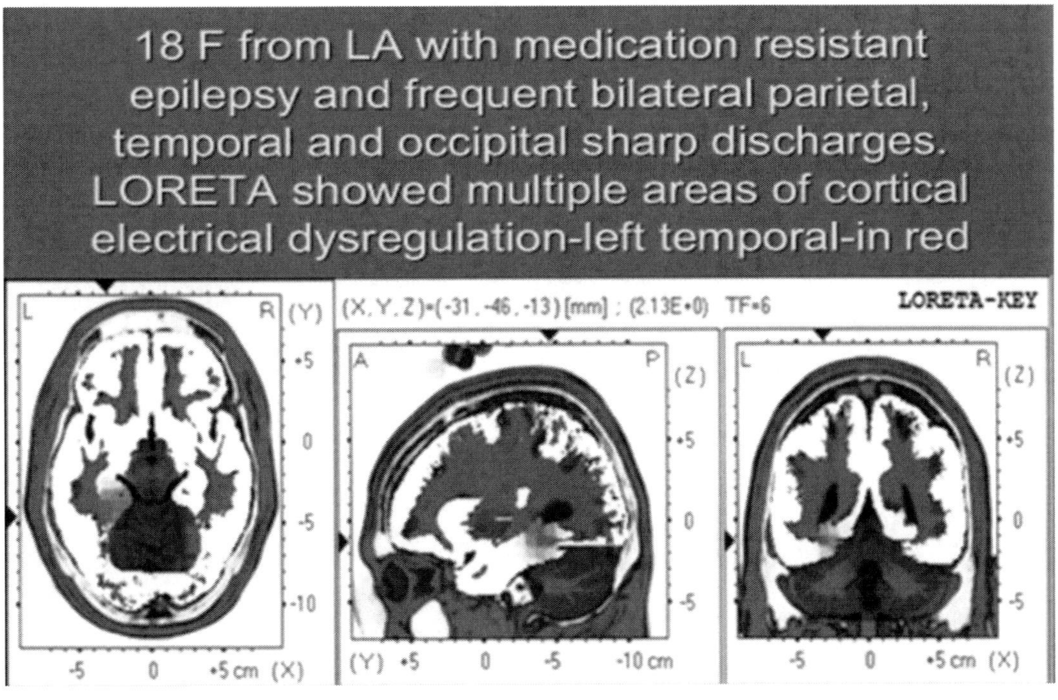

Figure 14. LORETA imaging before NFB initiation-only one of many areas of cortical dysregulations is shown (areas in red).

Prior to NFB, she was treated with Electro-Convulsive Therapy (ECT), which was not successful in relieving her depression. Instead, the individual sustained major memory impairment and visual-spatial difficulties. Since she was not responding to conventional therapy, her psychiatrist referred her to my practice for NFB therapy. The patient's cognitive and depressive dysfunction caused inability to continue her employment as a pharmaceutical representative. Initial LORETA showed several areas of electrical dysregulation including (Figure 15 A) BA-5 (secondary sensorimotor cortex), BA-9 (prefrontal cortex) and temporal cortex (not shown).

Her computerized cognitive testing before NFB showed deficiency in memory, information processing speed and visual-spatial domains (Figure 16). After 10 sessions of Z-score LORETA NFB, the patient reported major improvement in her mood (as well as mild memory improvement). Repeated computerized cognitive testing revealed marked improvement of previously deficient cognitive domains (Figure 16). Memory score increased from 85.4 to 102.8, information processing speed rose from 90.8 to 97.7 and visual-spatial domain went up from 80.8 to 100.7. In addition, post NFB LORETA showed an improvement of previously identified electrical dysregulation (Figure 15 B). After successful NFB therapy, the patient also was able to come back to gainful employment in the medical field (after a few years of being unemployed).

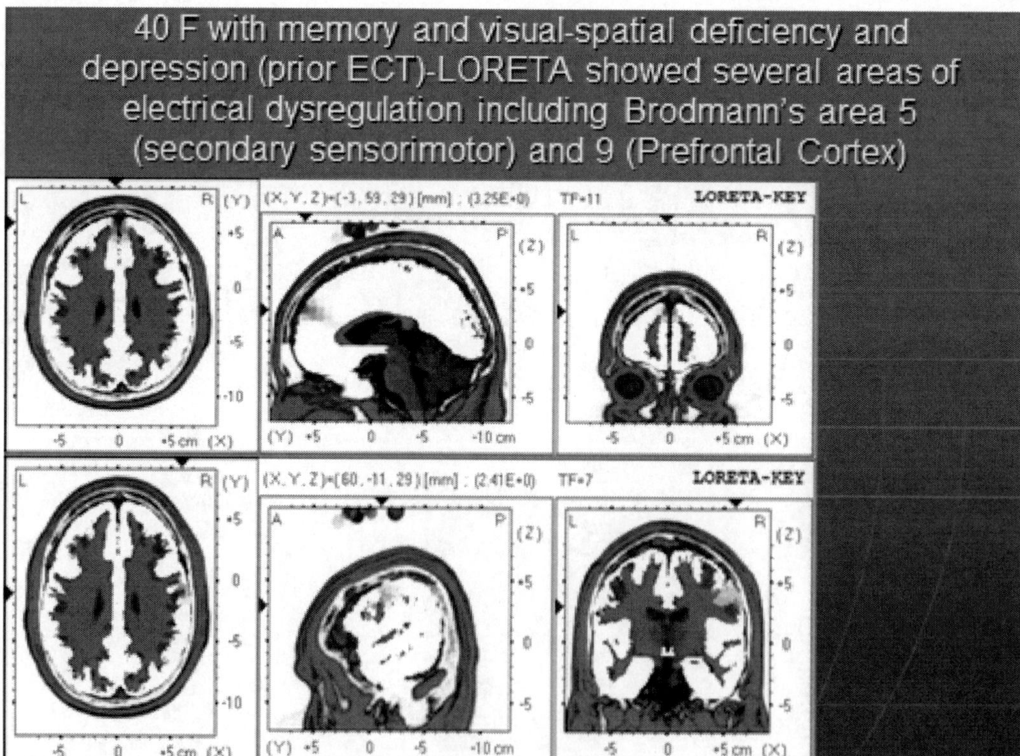

Figure 15 B. (Continued).

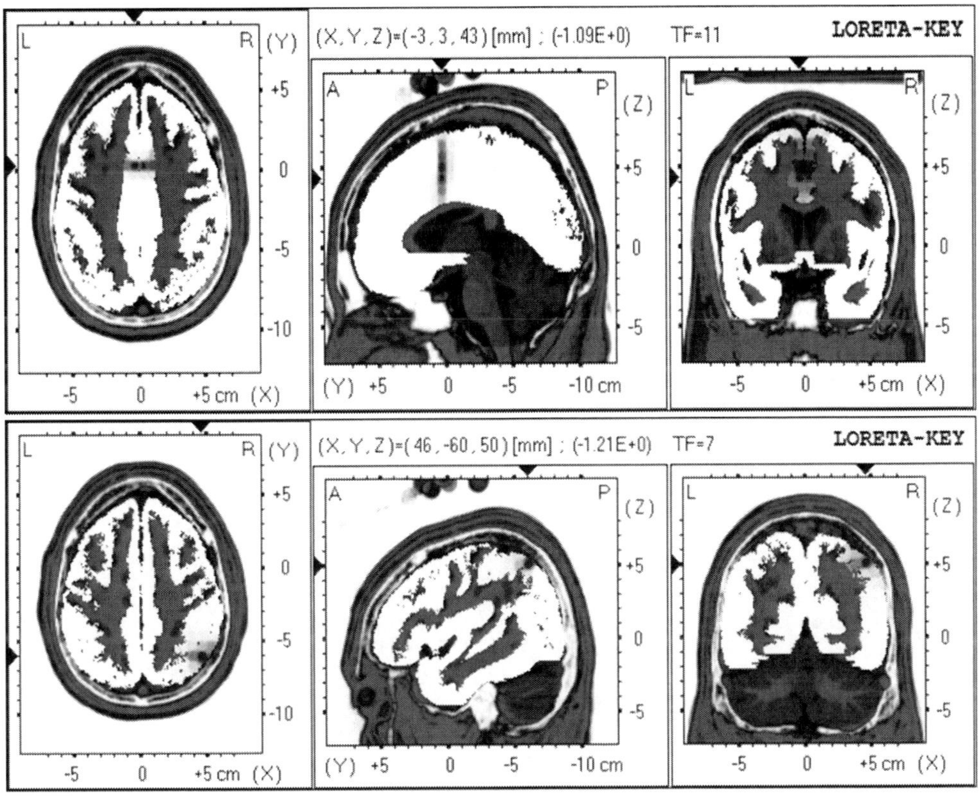

Figure 15 B. -40 year old female-LORETA after NFB-shows resolution of previously electrically dysregulated BA-5 and BA-9.

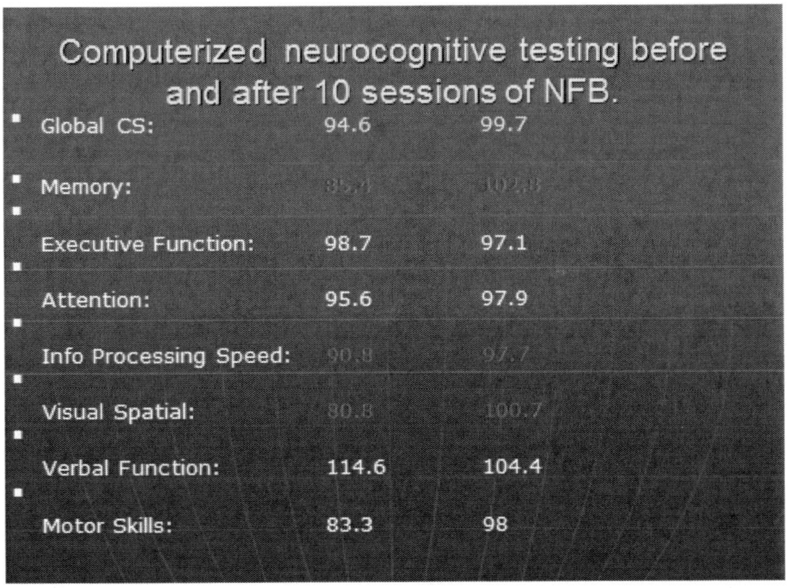

Figure 16. First vertical row shows scores from computerized cognitive testing before NFB. Second vertical row shows scores after 10 sessions of NFB. Computerized cognitive testing (Neurotrax Corp, Bellaire TX) shows data based on comparison to age and education matched controls. Expected score is 100 with 1 standard deviation being- 15.

Case 8

58 year old university professor was seen in my office due to major depression associated with anxiety and memory problems. She noticed problems with teaching due to possible cognitive dysfunction. Figure 17 shows her LORETA imaging before NFB, which identified several areas of electrical dysregulation including the cingulate cortex and left temporal region.

The computerized cognitive testing completed before NFB identified deficiency of memory and executive function. Blood work was negative for B12 deficiency.

After 10 sessions of NFB, major improvement in memory (from 42.8 to 107.1) was recorded on neurocognitive testing (Figure 18). In addition, marked improvement in the patient's mood and anxiety was reported. Post-NFB LORETA imaging confirmed an improvement in electrical dysregulation of previously identified regions (picture not shown). Patient also reported better performance in her academic settings.

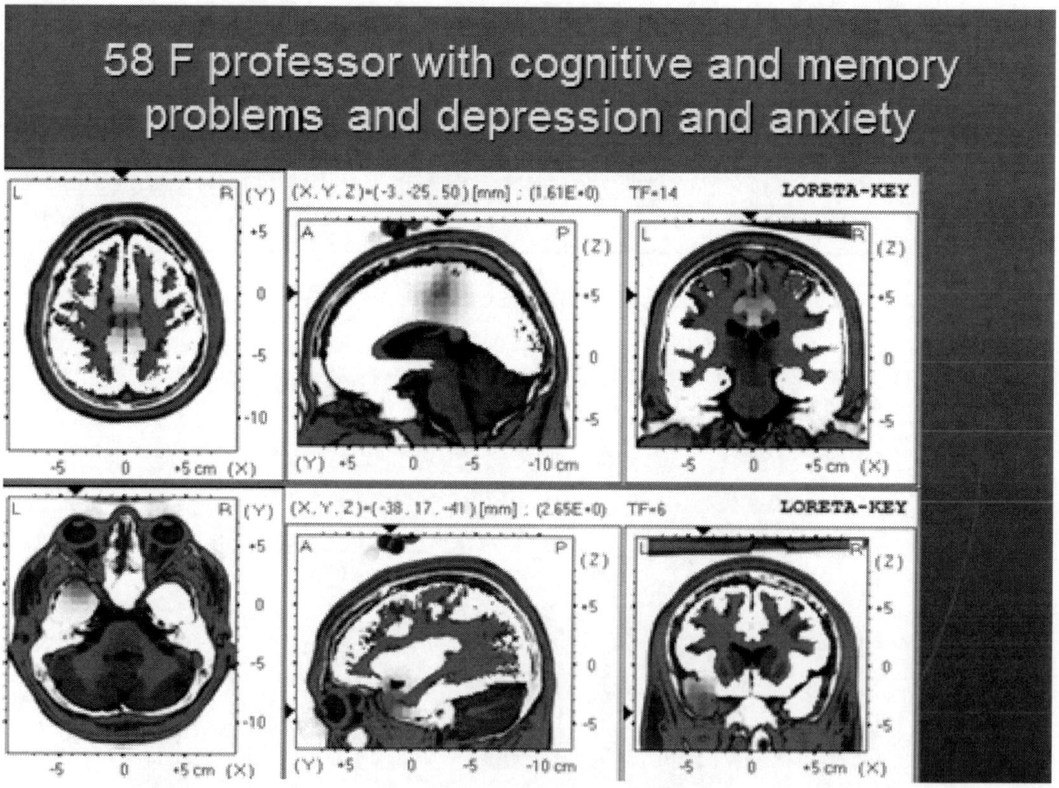

Figure 17. 58 year old female-LORETA imaging before NFB shows two areas of electrical dysregulation (in red) including the cingulate cortex and left temporal region.

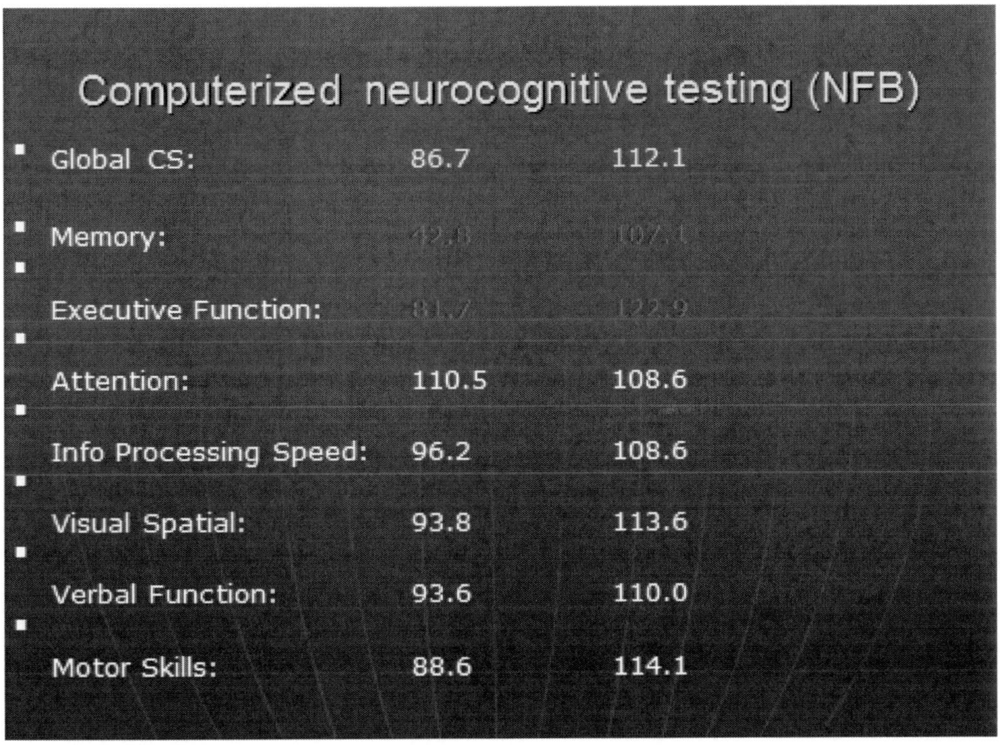

Figure 18. 58 year old female cognitive testing results before (left column) and after (right column) 10 sessions of NFB. Expected score is 100 with 1 standard deviation-15.

My clinic has already reported evidence of successful cognitive enhancement (Koberda, Moses, Koberda, Koberda, 2012 and Koberda, 2012) with LORETA Z-score NFB. One case report included an individual with Asperger's Syndrome (Koberda, 2012) associated with speech expressive dysfunction; another one described a student with low information processing speed and decreased memory (Koberda, Moses, Koberda, Koberda, 2012). Subsequently we have conducted a larger case series report where 35 consecutive patients complaining of cognitive dysfunction were subjected to LORETA Z-score NFB therapy (Koberda, Moses A, Koberda P, Winslow J, 2014). Before NFB initiation, these patients were evaluated with computerized neurocognitive testing in order to document and confirm any cognitive dysfunction reported in chief complaint. Many patients underwent brain imaging and laboratory testing to rule out any treatable condition which could have contributed to the patient's symptoms. Electrical imaging with QEEG/LORETA localization was also completed in order to visualize any area of cortical electrical dysregulation which could have been potentially responsible for the patient's symptoms (with specific Brodmann's Areas). The NFB protocol was based either on the patient's symptoms, the area of cortical dysregulation, or both. After 10 sessions of surface/LORETA Z-score NFB, the computerized cognitive testing and QEEG were repeated in order to see if any increase in cognitive score and/or reduction in QEEG abnormalities were achieved. In addition, the subjective patient's response was recorded as to whether or not they felt that the therapy was beneficial. Twenty-five patients (71%) were identified as of having a significant objective improvement (on average 10 points) through in cognitive testing. In addition, the subjective cognitive improvement and an objective reduction of QEEG abnormalities with NFB were also achieved in most of the patients. These results are very promising and indicate good effectiveness of LORETA Z-score NFB in cognitive enhancement.

This clinical data illustrates high effectiveness of Z-score LORETA NFB therapy in complex neuropsychiatric patients, where an improvement of pain, seizures, depression/anxiety and other associated cognitive domains can be achieved in most of the patients within just 10 treatment sessions. However, many patients requested to continue NFB for a longer period of time in order to continue benefits of this therapy.

Conclusion

This chapter illustrates diverse range of neuropsychiatric conditions which were identified as having significantly electrically dysregulated areas of the cortex by QEEG/LORETA technique. These cortical areas were specifically involved in regulation of functions which were affected by their illness/peak performance constraint. Z-score LORETA NFB is a modern biofeedback modality which may be used to correct these electrical abnormalities, and at the same time ameliorate patient's symptoms.

References

Billeci L, Sicca F, Maharatna K, Apicella F, Narzisi A, Campatelli G, Calderoni S, Pioggia G, Muratori F. On the application of quantitative EEG for characterizing autistic brain: a systematic review. *Front Hum. Neurosci*. 2013 Aug 5; 7:442.

Brett M, Johnsrude IS, Owen AM. The problem of functional localization in the human brain. *Nat. Rev. Neurosci*. 2002; 3(3):243–249.

Brunet E, Sarfati Y, Hardy-Baylé MC, Decety J. A PET investigation of the attribution of intentions with a nonverbal task. *Neuroimage*. 2000 Feb; 11(2):157-66.

Haas, L. F. (2003). "Hans Berger (1873-1941), Richard Caton (1842-1926), and electroencephalography". *Journal of Neurology, Neurosurgery & Psychiatry* 74 (1): 9. doi:10.1136/jnnp.74.1.9. PMC 1738204. PMID 12486257.

Koberda J. L. Moses A, Koberda P, Koberda L. (2013). Clinical advantages of quantitative electroencephalogram (QEEG)-electrical neuroimaging application in general neurology practice-Clin. *EEG Neurosci*. Oct; 44(4):273-85.

Koberda J. L. (2012). Autistic Spectrum Disorder (ASD) as a Potential Target of Z-score LORETA Neurofeedback. Neuroconnection- winter 2012, edition (ISNR), p. 24.

Koberda JL, Koberda P, Bienkiewicz A, Moses A, Koberda L. Pain Management Using 19-Electrode Z-Score LORETA Neurofeedback. *Journal of Neurotherapy*, 2013, 17:3, 179-190.

Koberda JL, Moses A, Koberda P, Winslow J. Cognitive Enhancement with LORETA Z-score Neurofeedback. AAPB meeting, March, 2014.

Koberda JL, Moses A, Koberda P, Winslow J. Koberda L, Bienkiewicz A. Z-score LORETA Neurofeedback as a Potential Therapy in Depression/Anxiety and Cognitive Dysfunction. Neuroconnection-Summer 2014, p.52.

Koberda J. L., Moses A., Koberda L., Koberda P. (2012). Cognitive Enhancement Using 19-electrode Z-score Neurofeedback. *Journal of Neurotherapy*-3, 224-230.

Kübler A1, Dixon V, Garavan H. Automaticity and reestablishment of executive control-an fMRI study. *J. Cogn. Neurosci.* 2006 Aug;18(8):1331-42.

Lancaster JL, Woldorff MG, Parsons LM, Liotti M, Freitas CS, Rainey L, Kochunov PV, Nickerson D, Mikiten SA, Fox PT. Automated Talairach Atlas labels for functional brain mapping. *Human Brain Mapping*. 2000; 10(3):120–131. doi: 10.1002/1097-0193(200007)10:3<120::AID-HBM30>3.0.CO;2-8. [PubMed] [Cross Ref]

Logothetis NK, Pauls J, Augath M, Trinath T, Oeltermann A. Neurophysiological investigation of the basis of the fMRI signal. *Nature*. 2001;412(6843):150–157.

Mazziotta J, Toga A, Evans A, Fox P, Lancaster J, Zilles K, Woods R, Paus T, Simpson G, Pike B. A probabilistic atlas and reference system for the human brain: International Consortium for Brain Mapping (ICBM) *Philosophical Transactions of the Royal Society of London Series B: Biological Sciences*. 2001; 356(1412):1293–1322.

Niedermeyer E. and da Silva F.L. (2004). Electroencephalography: Basic Principles, Clinical Applications, and Related Fields. Lippincot Williams & Wilkins. ISBN 0-7817-5126-8.

Nuwer, M. (1997). Assessment of digital EEG, quantitative EEG, and EEG brain mapping: report of the American Academy of Neurology and the American Clinical Neurophysiology Society. *Neurology* 49, 277–292.

Nunez PL, Srinivasan R (1981). Electric fields of the brain: The neurophysics of EEG. Oxford University Press.

Nunez, P. L., Srinivasan, R., Douglas Fields, R., EEG functional connectivity, axon delays and white matter disease, *Clinical Neurophysiology* (2014) in press.

Pascual-Marqui RD, Michel CM, Lehmann D. Low resolution electromagnetic tomography: a new method for localizing electrical activity in the brain. *Int. J. Psychophysiol.* 1994; 18(1):49–65. doi: 10.1016/0167-8760(84)90014-X. [PubMed] [Cross Ref]

Pizzagalli D, Pascual-Marqui RD, Nitschke JB, Oakes TR, Larson CL, Abercrombie HC, Schaefer SM, Koger JV, Benca RM, Davidson RJ. Anterior cingulate activity as a predictor of degree of treatment response in major depression: evidence from brain electrical tomography analysis. *Am. J. Psychiatry*. 2001;158(3):405–415. doi: 10.1176/appi.ajp.158.3.405. [PubMed] [Cross Ref].

Shmuel A, Augath M, Oeltermann A, Logothetis NK. Negative functional MRI response correlates with decreases in neuronal activity in monkey visual area V1. *Nature Neuroscience*. 2006;9(4):569–577.

Sitaram R, Caria A, Veit R, Gaber T, Rota G, Kuebler A, Birbaumer N. FMRI brain-computer interface: a tool for neuroscientific research and treatment. *Comput. Intell. Neurosci.* 2007:25487. doi: 10.1155/2007/25487.

Thatcher RW. Handbook of QEEG and EEG Biofeedback. (2012). Electronic edition.

Thatcher RW. (2013). Latest developments in live z-score training: Symptom checklist, phase reset, and LORETA z-score biofeedback. *Journal of Neurotherapy*, 17, 69–87.

Zhang JX1, Leung HC, Johnson MK. Frontal activations associated with accessing and evaluating information in working memory: an fMRI study. *Neuroimage*. 2003 Nov; 20(3):1531-9.

Zumsteg D, Friedman A, Wieser HG, Wennberg RA. Propagation of interictal discharges in temporal lobe epilepsy: Correlation of spatiotemporal mapping with intracranial foramen ovale electrode recordings. *Clinical Neurophysiology*. 2006; 117(12):2615–2626.

Young KD, Zotev V, Phillips R, Misaki M, Yuan H, Drevets WC, Bodurka J. Real-time FMRI neurofeedback training of amygdala activity in patients with major depressive disorder. *PLoS One*. 2014 Feb 11;9(2):e88785. doi: 10.1371/journal.pone.0088785. eCollection 2014.

In: Advances in Neuroimaging Research
Editor: Victoria Asher-Hansley
ISBN: 978-1-63321-307-4

Chapter III

Prenatal Magnetic Resonance Imaging of the Brain and Spine: Current Concepts, Advances and Future

F. C. G. Pinto[1] ***and M. F. Oliveira***[2*]

[1]Division of Functional Neurosurgery of the Institute of Psychiatry, Hospital das Clínicas, Universidade de São Paulo, São Paulo, Brazil

[2]Department of Neurosurgery - Hospital do Servidor Público Estadual de São Paulo, São Paulo-Brazil

Abstract

Fetal magnetic resonance (MR) imaging is an increasingly available technique used to evaluate the fetal brain and spine. This has become possible due to recent advances in technology and advances in coil design, making this diagnostic tool applicable in pregnant women with low risks to the mother and fetus. This provides a unique opportunity to evaluate processes that cannot be approached by any other current imaging technique and affords a unique opportunity for studying in vivo brain development and early diagnosis of congenital abnormalities inadequately visualized or undetectable by prenatal sonography. We discuss briefly about technical features like utility, application and safety and focus mainly on normal fetal brain development, role of fetal MR imaging in the evaluation of fetal ventriculomegaly, brain abnormalities such as of the corpus callosum, malformations of cortical development and spine abnormalities, such as spinal dysraphism. We present the medical and economical impact of such diagnostic modality and also discuss some challenges and advances towards future outcomes.

* Corresponding author: Matheus Fernandes de Oliveira; mafernoliv@yahoo.com.br; Av. Pedro de Toledo, 1800 – Vila Clementino, São Paulo – São Paulo – Brazil.

Introduction

Fetal magnetic resonance (MR) imaging is an increasingly available technique used to evaluate the fetal brain and spine. This has become possible due to recent advances in technology and advances in coil design, making this diagnostic tool applicable in pregnant women with lower risks to the mother and fetus [1,2,3,4].

The development of an ultrafast T2-weighted technique (known as *single-shot fast spin echo* and *half-Fourier acquisition turbo spin-echo*) has contributed to the increasing clinical use of fetal MR imaging, with protocols which take less than 1 second for image acquisition [5,6,7].

Fetal MR imaging allows direct visualization of the developing brain parenchyma, is not susceptible to the same limitations as ultrasound, and has higher contrast resolution than prenatal ultrasound, thereby allowing better differentiation of normal from abnormal tissue. Structural abnormalities, such as cerebral malformations and destructive lesions, can be sonographically occult on prenatal ultrasound yet detectable by fetal MR imaging [5,6,7,8].

Moreover, fetal MR imaging offers the promise of contributing to our understanding of normal as well as abnormal brain development with continued advances in MR imaging techniques, such as diffusion- weighted and parallel imaging [9,10,11,12].

Indications

Fetal MR imaging is essentially used for better characterization of abnormalities detected by routine prenatal sonography. Once it is more expensive and with less availability, screening tests are still performed by sonography [13,14,15,16,17].

The most common referral diagnose for fetal MR imaging is ventriculomegaly. Other common indications include sonographically suspected abnormalities of the corpus callosum and cerebellar vermis, patients with a history of a prior child or fetus with CNS anomalies or a genetic disorder. In these cases, fetal MR imaging is performed even when the prenatal sonogram is normal, because brain malformations can be difficult to detect with sonography [13,14,15,16,17].

Fetal MR imaging may also be used to evaluate brain and spine in cases of twin-twin transfusion syndrome and cotwin demise. Additional indications for fetal MR imaging include maternal illness, such as a maternal infection or major cardiac event [16,17,18,19,20].

Table 1. Common indications for fetal neuroimaging

Ventriculomegaly
Suspected malformation
Potential destructive lesion
Multiple malformations in the fetus
Malformation in siblings/known family history of genetic disease
Maternal infection

Safety of Fetal MR Imaging

Although application of fetal MR imaging is quite recent (mid- 1980s), there has been no consistent evidence to suggest harmful effects from short term exposure of the fetus to changing electromagnetic fields. Few animal experiments revealed no harmful events of fetal MRI, however it is still early to extrapolate such results to humans [15,16,17,18,20].

MR imaging is accepted as a safe and valuable imaging tool in prenatal evaluation of the fetus. However, MR imaging should not be performed in the first trimester of organogenesis, but can be safely performed from 18 weeks onwards. Field strength of up to 1.5 Tesla may be used [15,16,17,18,20].

Advantages of Fetal MR Imaging

Fetal MR imaging has several advantages over prenatal ultrasound, including improved contrast resolution. In addition, fetal MR imaging is able to visualize both sides of the developing brain directly. This is an advantage over ultrasound, where the ‘‘up-side’’ hemisphere is often shadowed by overlying structures, resulting in visualization of only the ‘‘down-side’’ hemisphere [15,16,17,18,20].

Other limitations of ultrasound, such as decreased amniotic fluid volume, fetal positioning, and shadowing from the bony calvarium, can also be overcome by fetal MR imaging. Thus, fetal MR imaging allows a more detailed evaluation of the developing brain, including direct visualization and assessment of the developing cortex and sulcation pattern, which is extremely difficult and often not possible with ultrasound [15,16,17,18,20].

MR imaging can detect sonographically occult abnormalities in up to 50% of cases. These sonographically occult abnormalities include developmental and destructive lesions, such as agenesis of the corpus callosum, cortical malformation, periventricular nodular heterotopia, cerebellar dysplasia, periventricular leukomalacia, porencephaly, multicystic encephalomalacia, germinal matrix hemorrhage, and intraventricular hemorrhage [15,16,17,18,20].

Table 2. Comparison of antenatal use of ultrasound and magnetic resonance

Ultrasound	Magnetic resonance
Cheap	Expensive
Real time method	High resolution study
Doppler evaluation	Hemorrhage and fat can be viewed in T1
Applicable in throughout gestation	Functional studies
Padronization of anatomic reference points	Spectroscopy
Vulnerability to mother obesity	Not applicable in first trimester
Less quality in Oligoamnion	Lack of study standardization
Lower resolution	Fetal movement
Posterior shadow	Claustrophoby

MR Imaging Techniques

Fetal MR imaging is routinely performed on 1.5-T scanners. There are several limitations to fetal MR imaging, including fetal motion, the small size of the structure being imaged (particularly at younger gestational ages), and the distance between the receiver coil and the structure being imaged [1,2,3,4,5,15,16,17,18,20].

When performing fetal MR imaging, sedating agents are not administered during the examination. Intravenous contrast is also not recommended in fetal MR imaging because of the potential risk to the fetus [15,16,17,18,20].

The mother lies supine during the course of the examination, which typically lasts 45 minutes. If the mother cannot tolerate lying on her back (e.g., because of back pain or compression of the inferior vena cava), the examination can be performed with the mother lying on her left side. To reduce fetal motion, the mother is instructed not to eat or drink anything for 4 hours before the MR imaging examination [15,16,17,18,20].

For imaging the fetal brain, ssFSE T2-weighted images are obtained using a slice thickness of 3 mm with no gap. For the fetal spine, a 2-mm slice thickness is used. Images are acquired during free maternal breathing, although we have found respiratory gating useful to decrease motion. The field of view is typically small, although this should be adjusted for increased fetal or maternal size or when aliasing artifact is problematic [15,16,17,18,20].

The application of T1-weighed imaging to fetal MR imaging is more limited. This sequence yields eight slices in the axial plane. Images are acquired during a single maternal breath hold. Alternative T1-weighted techniques are being explored but are still subject to the limitations of the long T1 relaxation time of the fetal brain [15,16,17,18,20]. Advanced MR imaging techniques, such as diffusion-weighted imaging, spectroscopy, and parallel imaging have also recently been successfully applied to fetal MR imaging. Diffusion weighted imaging provides quantitative information about water motion and tissue microstructure. Fetal diffusion-weighted imaging has applications for developmental and destructive brain processes [15,16,17,18,20].

Because of the long acquisition time (4.5 minutes) and size of the voxel relative to the small size of the fetal brain, MR spectroscopy is currently limited in its application to pregnancies in the third trimester. Shorter acquisition times can be used, although they are limited by signal to noise [15,16,17,18,20].

Normal metabolites, such as N-acetylaspartate, creatine, and choline, can be detected in fetuses of advanced gestational age. Parallel imaging can also be applied to fetal MR imaging to decrease the scan time, increase image resolution, or decrease the specific absorption rate [15,16,17,18,20].

Fetal MR Clinical Applications of Fetal MR Imaging

Ventriculomegaly

Ventriculomegaly is the most common CNS abnormality identified on prenatal sonography (Figure 1 and 2). It is defined as atrial width greater than 10 mm on a sonogram.

The etiologies of ventriculomegaly are heterogeneous and include developmental, destructive, and obstructive processes [8,9,10,11,12,13,14].

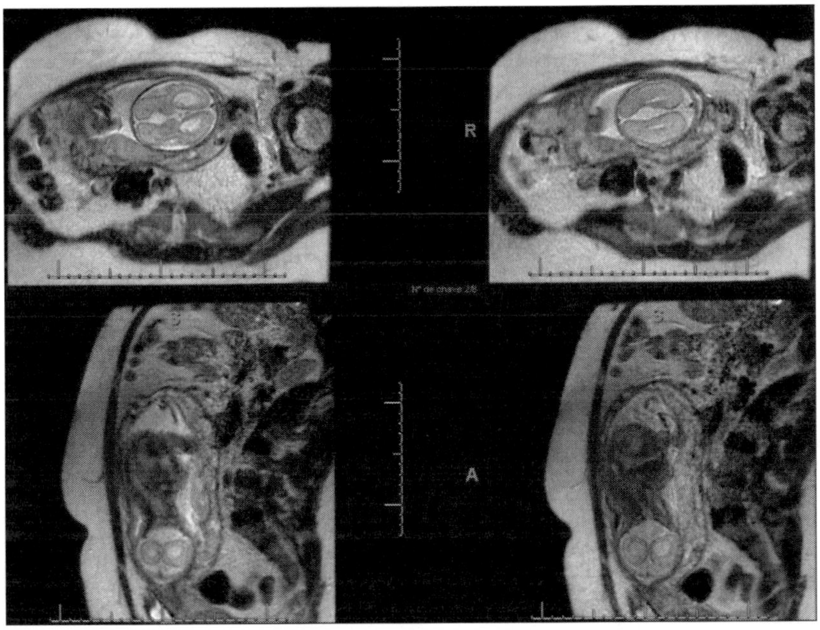

Figure 1. Example of ventriculomegaly identified by antenatal MR, with interhemispheric cyst.

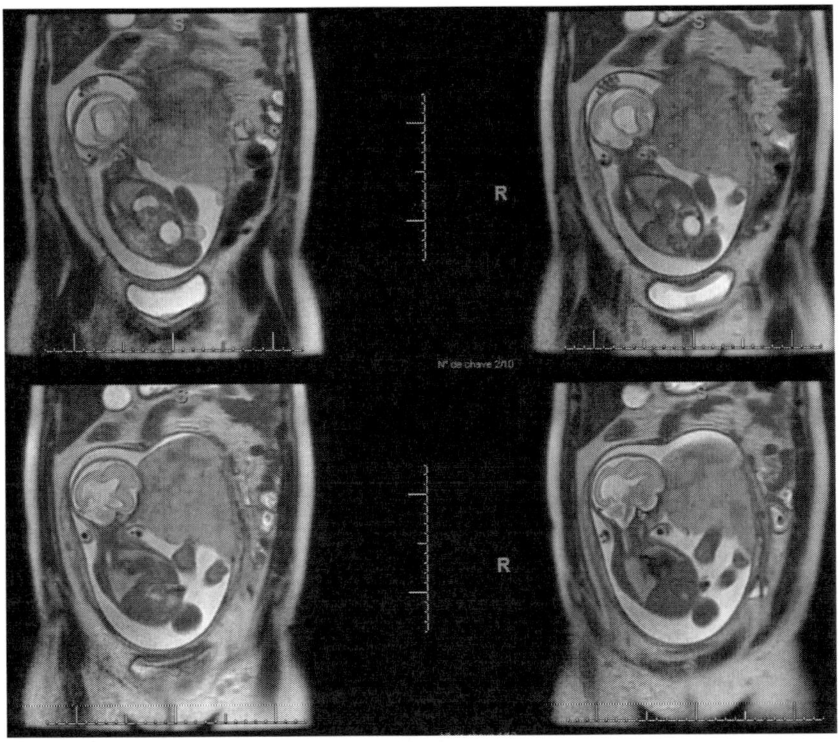

Figure 2. Ventriculomegaly with lissencephaly.

Additional abnormalities have been reported in up to 80% of fetuses with ventriculomegaly and include CNS, extra- CNS, and chromosomal anomalies. Neural tube defects, agenesis of the corpus callosum, Dandy- Walker malformation, lissencephaly, holoprosencephaly (Figure 3), gray matter heterotopia, polymicrogyria, intraventricular hemorrhage, subependymal hemorrhage. and porencephaly have been described in association with ventriculomegaly. Studies on the neurodevelopmental outcome of prenatally diagnosed ventriculomegaly have shown a better prognosis when it is an isolated finding [8,9,10,11,12,13,14].

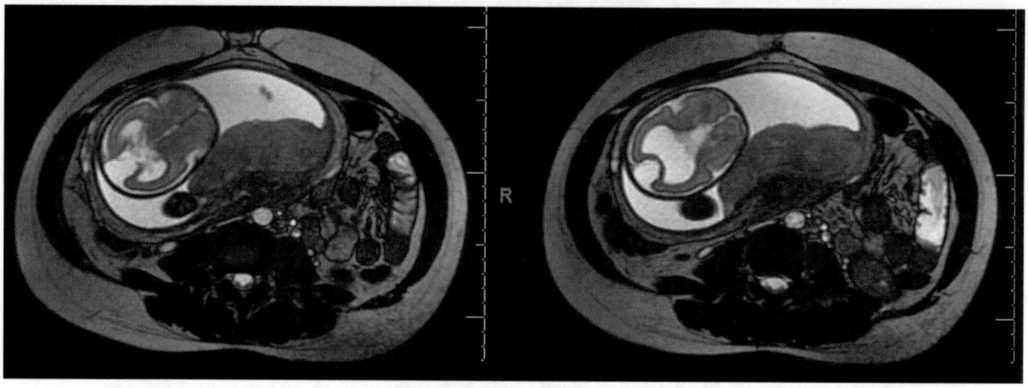

Figure 3. Holoprosencephaly.

Hemorrhage

Hemorrhage is usually detected as areas of hypointensity on T2-weighted images or hyperintensity on T1-weighted images, although the signal intensity can vary depending on the stage of hemorrhage. Hemorrhage can occur within the ventricle, appearing as debris layering within the ventricle or as a focal hematoma, or within the adjacent brain parenchyma. We have found detection of small subependymal hemorrhage to be more difficult because the germinal matrix is normally hypointense on T2-weighted images and hyperintense on T1-weighted images because of its high cellularity [8,9,10,11,12,13,14].

Ischemia/Infarction

Fetal MR imaging is the preferred modality to demonstrate fetal ischemia or infarction. This may not be apparent by US. Diffusion-weighted imaging can further aid in demonstration of acute to subacute ischemic lesions.14 The classic ischemia of arterial distribution is not the common pattern seen in utero. Ischemia in the fetal brain may involve the cortical ribbon and white matter or just the white matter alone [8,9,10,11,12,13,14].

Hemorrhagic infarction is more common. Ischemic cerebral changes in utero may result in white matter necrosis or leukomalacia. On fetal MR imaging, particular attention should be paid to the morphology of the germinal matrix to identify presence of any focal areas of T2 hypointensity or increased susceptibility on gradient images [15,16,17,18,20].

Vascular Malformations

Intracranial vascular malformations are rare in the fetus or neonate but when present are usually symptomatic high-flow lesions. High-flow vascular malformations are comprised of abnormal connections between arteries and veins in which the arteries either communicate directly with a draining vein through a macroscopic fistula (arteriovenous fistula) or through an interposed vascular nidus (arteriovenous malformation) [15,16,17,18,20].

Arteriovenous shunting may produce in utero congestive heart failure, fetal hydrops, hydrocephalus, and ischemic brain injury. High-flow malformations may develop within the dura, subarachnoid space, or brain parenchyma. Both dural and subarachnoid spaces are occasionally evaluated with fetal MR imaging. Parenchymal vascular malformations rarely present in the neonate and have not been reported using obstetric MR imaging [15,16,17,18,20].

Vein of Galen Malformation

The most common cerebrovascular malformation diagnosed in prenatal life is the Galen vein malformation. The pathophysiology of this lesion is abnormal communication of arterial feeders from the circle of Willis as well as the vertebrobasilar arterial system, which anastomose with the galenic venous system, which then becomes aneurysmally dilated [15,16,17,18,20]. There is usually accompanying cardiomegaly and high-output congestive heart failure. Cerebral ischemic lesions may occur due to steal phenomenon. When there is obstruction of the venous outflow, hydrocephalus may be present. Prenatal MR evaluation can delineate the abnormally enlarged vessels and the dilated Galen vein. In addition, MR imaging can also identify the cerebral ischemic lesions and hemorrhage as well as hydrocephalus that may also be present [15,16,17,18,20].

Anomalies of the Fetal Face and Skull

Anomalies of the fetal face, skull, and neck may be observed as isolated abnormalities. When these abnormalities are detected on US, the role of MR imaging is to detect any associated abnormalities of the brain. More commonly, fetal face, skull, and neck anomalies are visualized in association with CNS abnormalities, chromosomal abnormalities, and syndromes [15,16,17,18,20].

Orbit Abnormalities

Hypotelorism is defined as decrease in the normal intraocular distance below the fifth percentile for gestational age. Typically, hypotelorism is commonly associated with midline malformations of the brain, such as holoprosencephaly. It can also occur with other chromosomal abnormalities, syndromes, and abnormal calvarial development. Hypertelorism is defined as increased interocular distance or abnormally wide-set eyes. Hypertelorism may be an isolated abnormality. Hypertelorism is known to occur with anterior cephalocele due to mechanical disruption of migration of the orbits from a lateral to a more anterior position [15,16,17,18,20].

Cleft Lip and Palate

Cleft lip may occur in isolation or with cleft palate and could be unilateral or bilateral defect. The defect is usually well identified on MR as amniotic fluid filling the cleft. When the cleft is complete, it extends from the upper lip to the nose and the hard palate. Closely apposed clefts, however, may be difficult to be visualized on MR. When the cleft is complete and bilateral, it is usually associated with elevation of the median nasal prominence and characteristic premaxillary protrusion [15,16,17,18,20].

Mandibular Abnormalities

A small or receding mandible (retrognathia) may result in micrognathia. Micrognathia and retrognathia are associated with multiple syndromes and chromosomal abnormalities. Pierre Robin syndrome is one such complex abnormality that is characterized by severe mandibular hypoplasia. Consequent to a small mandible, the size of the oral cavity is significantly reduced with a normalsized tongue falling back and resulting in airway obstruction. This abnormality can result in the fetus unable to swallow adequately and has significant hazard for airway obstruction.33 There is associated polyhydramnios. Similar to fetuses with large facial and cervical masses, which have potential for the fetal airway to be obstructed, fetuses with severe mandibular hypoplasia have risk for airway obstruction. Abnormalities of the fetal skull shape can occur due to several causes, such as hydrocephalus [15,16,17,18,20].

Abnormalities of the Corpus Callosum

Abnormalities of the corpus callosum consist of agenesis, hypogenesis (or partial agenesis), dysgenesis, hypoplasia, and destruction. The exact incidence of callosal agenesis is not known. It has been estimated at 0.2% to 0.7% in the general population and 3% in mentally disabled patients [15,16,17,18,20].

Although callosal agenesis has been reported as an incidental finding, patients can have variable neurologic symptoms, including developmental delay, mental disability, and epilepsy. Callosal anomalies are highly associated with other CNS anomalies as well as with specific syndromes, such as Aicardi syndrome. On autopsy, 85% of patients with callosal agenesis have additional CNS anomalies and 62% have additional extra-CNS anomalies. The detection of associated anomalies is significant in that these patients tend to have a higher incidence of motor or mental disabilities [15,16,17,18,20].

Callosal anomalies can be difficult to detect on ultrasound, particularly in late gestation or when the fetal head is engaged in the maternal pelvis. Fetal MR imaging is useful in the evaluation of suspected callosal anomalies because (1) the corpus callosum can be directly visualized in the sagittal and coronal planes after 20 weeks and (2) associated anomalies are more easily detected as compared with ultrasound. Fetal MR imaging has been reported to identify an intact corpus callosum in approximately 20% of cases referred for sonographically suspected callosal abnormalities, which has significant implications for patient counseling. Fetal MR imaging has also been reported to have greater detection of callosal agenesis as compared with prenatal ultrasound [15,16,17,18,20].

Posterior Fossa Abnormalities

Posterior fossa anomalies imaged with fetal MR imaging include Dandy-Walker malformation, Joubert syndrome, Dandy-Walker variant, mega cisterna magna, arachnoid cyst, Blake's pouch cyst, cerebellar dysplasia, cerebellar hypoplasia, cerebellar hemorrhage, and Chiari II malformation [15,16,17,18,20].

Dandy-Walker malformation refers to the occurrence of agenesis or hypoplasia of the vermis in association with an enlarged posterior fossa, elevated tentorium, and cystic dilatation fourth ventricle. More mild forms of vermian hypoplasia with a more normal posterior fossa have been referred to as the Dandy-Walker variant, although the terms Dandy-Walker and Dandy-Walker variant have at times been confused. In addition, Blake's pouch cyst has been referred to as being within the Dandy-Walker continuum. Although severe Dandy-Walker malformations can be fairly easily identified on ultrasound, it can be hard to distinguish more mild forms of vermian hypoplasia from a mega cisterna magna or an arachnoid cyst with a normal-appearing cerebellar vermis [15,16,17,18,20].

In addition, ossification of the skull can impede sonographic visualization of the posterior fossa in the third trimester. In these cases, fetal MR imaging can play an important diagnostic role. In particular, fetal MR imaging can be used to assess the shape and size of the vermis in cases of suspected vermian hypoplasia [15,16,17,18,20].

In addition, MR imaging can be helpful in evaluating the relation between a posterior fossa cyst and the fourth ventricle. Although only a limited number of posterior fossa abnormalities are reported in the fetal MR imaging literature, several authors have found fetal MR imaging to be helpful. When a Dandy-Walker malformation is confirmed, MR imaging can also be used to detect associated CNS abnormalities. These include agenesis of the corpus callosum, polymicrogyria, neuronal heterotopia, and occipital encephaloceles [15,16,17,18,20].

Fetal MR imaging is also helpful in evaluating posterior fossa echogenic masses. In these cases, it can be used to assess the integrity of the cerebellar hemispheres and vermis and to identify the location of the hemorrhage. Lesions evaluated by fetal MR imaging include cerebellar parenchymal hemorrhages and vascular malformations [15,16,17,18,20].

Complications of Monochorionic Twin Pregnancies

Fetal MR imaging can be used to identify parenchymal injury in monochorionic twin pregnancies, which are at increased risk for brain injury. Monochorionic twins share a common placenta that often contains abnormal intertwin vascular connections [15,16,17,18,20].

Fetal MR imaging can detect destructive parenchymal lesions, such as those that may result after the demise of a cotwin. Ischemic parenchymal injuries can manifest as focal or diffuse areas of increased T2 signal in the germinal matrix, developing white matter, or cortex. Furthermore, ischemic injury can also result in cortical malformations detectable by fetal MR imaging, such as polymicrogyria [15,16,17,18,20].

In general, we have found that ischemic related injuries are best visualized if imaging is performed at least 2 weeks after the presumed event. It is possible that with advances in fetal diffusionweighted imaging, such injuries may be able to be detected sooner [15,16,17,18,20].

Fetal MR imaging can be useful in assessing brain injury in twins affected by twin-twin transfusion syndrome, although scanning of the polyhydramniotic twin can be difficult because of excessive fetal motion [19,20,21].

Malformations of Cortical Development

We have found fetal MR imaging to be especially helpful in identifying malformations of cortical development in cases of sonographically isolated ventriculomegaly [13,14,15,16,17,18,20].

Because of its better soft tissue contrast and ability to visualize several aspects of normal brain maturation, fetal MR imaging has significantly contributed to the prenatal identification of malformations of cortical development. Studies have shown that fetal MR imaging can detect cortical malformations that are not identified on ultrasound. In a study of 20 fetuses with migrational disorders confirmed on postnatal imaging or autopsy, fetal MR imaging was superior to ultrasound in identifying schizencephaly, lissencephaly, polymicrogyria, and gray matter heterotopia [13,14,15,16,17,18,20].

The imaging appearance of cortical malformations can be similar to that in the child. Subependymal heterotopias appear as nodules along the ventricular walls and are similar in signal intensity to the germinal matrix and developing cortex. As mentioned earlier, they cannot be reliably distinguished from subependymal nodules seen in tuberous sclerosis. Schizencephaly appears as a gray matter–lined cleft extending from the ventricle to the subarachnoid space. Polymicrogyria appears as multiple abnormal infoldings of the developing cortex. Classic lissencephaly can be identified by the shallow appearance of the Sylvian fissures, absence of additional sulci for the expected gestational age of the fetus, absence of normal multilayered appearance of the brain [13,14,15,16,17,18,20].

Spinal Disorders

For spine anomalies, fetal MR imaging is particularly helpful. It can be used to detect underlying spinal cord anomalies, such as diastematomyelia and segmental spinal dysgenesis, which can be occult on prenatal sonography [21,22,23,24].

One of the more common fetal spinal anomalies detected by prenatal sonography is myelomeningocele (Figure 4). Myelomeningoceles are almost always seen in combination with a small posterior fossa and herniation of cerebellar tissue into the cervical subarachnoid space and are referred to as Chiari II malformations [21,22,23,24].

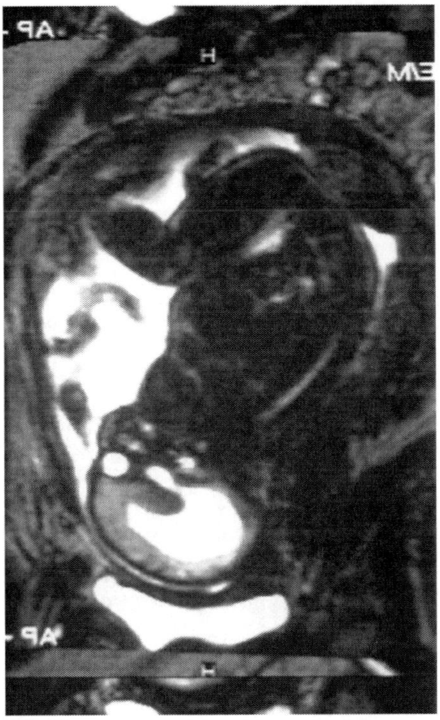

Figure 4. Typical case of Chiari II, with ventriculomegaly and lumbar myelomeningocele.

In general, Chiari II malformations and myelomeningoceles can be easily diagnosed on prenatal sonography. Fetal MR imaging can be helpful when ultrasound is limited, however, such as in cases of large maternal body habitus, oligohydramnios, low position of the fetal head, or when the fetal spine is positioned posteriorly with respect to the mother [21,22,23,24].

Fetal MR imaging is also useful in identifying additional CNS anomalies that are frequently associated with Chiari II malformations, such as callosal agenesis or hypogenesis, microgyria, polymicrogyria, periventricular nodular heterotopia, cerebellar dysplasia, syringohydromyelia, and diastematomyelia. The degree of hindbrain herniation and hydrocephalus as well as the severity of the spinal abnormality can also be evaluated with fetal MR imaging [21,22,23,24].

There has been an increasing trend towards the use of magnetic resonance imaging (MR) in prenatal fetal evaluation, as it is considered to provide better anatomical evaluation of the fetal spine and brain in myelomeningocele. Despite their increasing use, very few studies have tried to compare the accuracy of determining the level of spinal lesions by prenatal ultrasonography or antenatal MRI by correlation with the postnatal imaging and clinical findings [21,22,23,24].

The level of lesion has been shown to be the single most important outcome predictor of functional neurological outcome in spina bifida. Lower spinal lesions and smaller ventricular size are associated with better ambulatory status compared to high lesions and large ventricular size. Hence sonographic detection of lesion level and type is useful in predicting the ambulatory potential of fetuses with open spina bifida and helps counseling regarding the functional prognosis for this condition [21,22,23,24].

Future Advances in fetal MR Imaging

Fetal MRI is also used to study normal in utero brain development. This is important for establishing normative measures that can be used to better identify cases of abnormal brain development. Using fetal DWI, normative mean diffusivity values during the second and third trimesters have been established [15,16,17,18,20].

Because of the long acquisition time (several minutes) and size of the voxel relative to the fetal brain size, MR spectroscopy is limited to application in the third trimester when the fetal head is relatively large and engaged in the pelvis. Normal metabolites such as N-acetyl aspartate, creatine, choline, and myo-inositol can be detected, and several studies have shown changes in metabolite levels during gestation [15,16,17,18,20].

Functional MR studies have also recently been performed in fetuses during the third trimester and have primarily involved the application of an auditory stimulus to the maternal abdomen. These studies have shown temporal lobe activation in response to an auditory stimulus in some fetuses, as early as 33 gestational weeks [15,16,17,18,20].

An MR technique that has been described recently allows the noninvasive measurement of the oxygen partial pressure of fluids. This has been applied to the fetal cerebrospinal fluid. Because the oxygen content of cerebrospinal fluid can give information about the oxygenation of the surrounding cerebral tissues, this method might offer insight into conditions that result in decreased fetal cerebral oxygenation [15,16,17,18,20].

Although significant progress in the field of fetal MR imaging has occurred with the development of ultrafast T2-weighted techniques, continued technical advances are likely to contribute to significant growth of the field within the next few years. In particular, with the recent application of diffusion weighted imaging to the fetal brain, quantifiable aspects of brain development can now be studied noninvasively [15,16,17,18,20].

This has promising applications for the study of specific brain disorders as well as for the study of normal in utero brain development. Moreover, with continued hardware and software improvements, additional MR imaging sequences that are rapid, and therefore feasible to use in clinical practice, are likely to become available [15,16,17,18,20].

Because fetal MR imaging involves many disciplines, including physics, obstetrics, developmental neurobiology, genetics, perinatology, pediatric neurology, pediatric neurosurgery, and neuropathology, the future promise of fetal MR imaging is likely to be achieved through multidisciplinary collaborative efforts [15,16,17,18,20].

In practice, MR spectroscopy is usually performed after the standard magnetic resonance imaging (MRI) sequences. Acquisition time for a single spectroscopic sequence ranges from 2 to 7 min and the measurement of all necessary spectra usually takes up to 15 min. Short TE acquisition is used to detect metabolites with short spin–spin relaxation times, such as glutamine, glutamate, glucose, taurine and lipids. Resonances of *N* -acetyl aspartate (NAA), choline and creatine are also visible in short echo spectra, but due to their longer relaxation times their quantification is more accurate at longer TEs (135 and/or 270 ms) [15,16,17,18,20].

Conclusion

A multidisciplinary approach plays an important role in counseling expectant parents about fetal CNS malformations. Initially, the interaction of obstetricians, other specialist and parents may begin in the prenatal period to plan the timing and route of delivery. Postnatal management, including surgery, may be discussed in advance. Familiarity with imaging modalities will permit a better presentation of information for family counseling and decision making during and after the pregnancy.

Although ultrasonography has been the imaging method most commonly used for evaluating a fetus, MR imaging has proved to be a valuable complementary tool; it provides good anatomical and tissue definition for further characterization of an abnormality. Magnetic resonance imaging may also be beneficial in circumstances in which ultrasonography is technically limited.

References

[1] Hata T, Makihara K, Aoki S, Hata K, Kitao M. Magnetic resonance imaging of the fetus: initial experience. *Gynecol. Obstet. Invest.* 1990;29(4):255-8.

[2] Coakley FV, Glenn O, Payyum A, et al. Fetal MRI: a developing technique for the developing patient. *AJR Am. J. Roentgenol.* 2004;182:243–52.

[3] Raybaud C, Levrier O, Brunel H, et al. MR imaging of fetal brain malformations. *Childs Nerv. Syst.* 2003;19:455–70.

[4] Girard N, Raybaud C, Dercole C, et al. In vivo MRI of the fetal brain. *Neuroradiology* 1993; 35(6):431–6.

[5] Levine D, Barnes PD, Madsen JR, et al. Fetal CNS anomalies revealed on ultrafast MR imaging. *AJR Am. J. Roentgenol.* 1999;172(3):813–8.

[6] Glenn O, Goldstein R, Li K, et al. Fetal MRI in the evaluation of fetuses referred for sonographically suspected abnormalities of the cor- pus callosum. *J. Ultrasound Med.* 2005;24(6): 791–804.

[7] Whitby EH, Paley MNJ, Sprigg A, et al. Comparison of ultrasound and magnetic resonance imaging in 100 singleton pregnancies with suspected brain abnormalities. *BJOG: An International Journal of Obstetrics and Gynecology* 2004;111:784–92.

[8] Cavalheiro S, Moron AF, Almodin CG, Suriano IC, Hisaba V, Dastoli P, Barbosa MM. Fetal hydrocephalus. *Childs Nerv. Syst.* 2011 Oct;27(10):1575-83.

[9] Papadias A, Miller C, Martin WL, Kilby MD, Sgouros S. Comparison of prenatal and postnatal MRI findings in the evaluation of intrauterine CNS anomalies requiring postnatal neurosurgical treatment. *Childs Nerv. Syst.* 2008 Feb;24(2):185-92.

[10] Cavalheiro S, Moron AF, Zymberg ST, Dastoli P. Fetal hydrocephalus--prenatal treatment. *Childs Nerv Syst.* 2003 Aug;19(7-8):561-73.

[11] Mangels KJ, Tulipan N, Tsao LY, Alarcon J, Bruner JP. Fetal MRI in the evaluation of intrauterine myelomeningocele. *Childs Nerv Syst*. 2013 Oct;29(10):1905-14.
[12] Tortori-Donati P, Rossi A, Biancheri R, Cama A. Magnetic resonance imaging of spinal dysraphism. *Top Magn Reson Imaging*. 2001 Dec;12(6):375-409.
[13] Erdem G, Celik O, Hascalik S, Karakas HM, Alkan A, Firat AK. Diffusion-weighted imaging evaluation of subtle cerebral microstructural changes in intrauterine fetalhydrocephalus. *Magn Reson Imaging*. 2007 Dec;25(10):1417-22.
[14] Glenn OA. MR imaging of the fetal brain. Pediatr Radiol. 2010 Jan;40(1):68-81.
[15] Glenn OA. Fetal central nervous system MR imaging. *Neuroimaging Clin. N. Am*. 2006 Feb;16(1):1-17, vii. Review.
[16] Glenn OA, Barkovich AJ. Magnetic resonance imaging of the fetal brain and spine: an increasingly important tool in prenatal diagnosis, part 1. *AJNR Am. J. Neuroradiol.* 2006 Sep;27(8):1604-11. Review.
[17] Glenn OA, Barkovich J. Magnetic resonance imaging of the fetal brain and spine: an increasingly important tool in prenatal diagnosis: part 2. *AJNR Am. J. Neuroradiol.* 2006 Oct;27(9):1807-14. Review.
[18] Miller E, Ben-Sira L, Constantini S, Beni-Adani L. Impact of prenatal magnetic resonance imaging on postnatal neurosurgical treatment. *J. Neurosurg*. 2006 Sep;105(3 Suppl):203-9.
[19] Pugash D, Krssak M, Kulemann V, Prayer D. Magnetic resonance spectroscopy of the fetal brain. *Prenat Diagn*. 2009 Apr;29(4):434-41.
[20] Shekdar K, Feygin T. Fetal neuroimaging. Neuroimaging *Clin. N. Am*. 2011 Aug;21(3):677-703, ix.
[21] Barnewolt CE, Estroff JA. Sonography of the fetal central nervous system. *Neuroimaging Clin. N. Am*. 2004 May;14(2):255-71, viii.
[22] Kline-Fath BM, Calvo-Garcia MA. Prenatal imaging of congenital malformations of the brain. *Semin Ultrasound CT MR*. 2011 Jun;32(3):167-88.
[23] Ben-Sira L, Garel C, Malinger G, Constantini S. Prenatal diagnosis of spinal dysraphism.*Childs Nerv Syst*. 2013 Sep;29(9):1541-52.
[24] Sgouros S. Spinal dysraphism. *Childs Nerv. Syst*. 2013 Sep;29(9):1415-6.

In: Advances in Neuroimaging Research
Editor: Victoria Asher-Hansley

ISBN: 978-1-63321-307-4

Chapter IV

Normal Pressure Hydrocephalus: Neuroimaging As a Tool for Differential Diagnosis and Outcome Predictor

F. C. G. Pinto[1] and M. F. Oliveira[2*]

[1]Division of Functional Neurosurgery of the Institute of Psychiatry, Hospital das Clínicas, Universidade de São Paulo, São Paulo, Brazil
[2]Department of Neurosurgery -
Hospital do Servidor Público Estadual de São Paulo,
São Paulo-Brazil

Abstract

Normal pressure hydrocephalus (NPH) is a condition characterized by gait disturbance, dementia and/or urinary incontinence without causative disorders, as well as dilation of ventricular system due to disturbance of cerebrospinal fluid (CSF) circulation with normal CSF pressure and no secondary cause· It is a differential diagnosis for most of the dementia syndromes and occurs mainly in elderly populations. Neuroimaging is fundamental not only in affirming diagnosis with anatomical patterns, but also increasing evidence points to qualitative and quantitative measures which are important to perform differential diagnosis with simultaneous diseases like Alzheimer disease and vascular dementia. Magnetic resonance imaging (MRI) and functional neuroimaging techniques like Positron Emission Tomography (PET) and Single Photon Emission Tomography (SPECT) are being employed to evaluate cerebrospinal fluid biomarkers and periventricular hemodynamic parameters in order to better classify those patients and predict their response to provocative tests and to shunt procedures. We discuss the main current aspects and new protocols towards management of NPH.

* Corresponding author: Matheus Fernandes de Oliveira; mafernoliv@yahoo.com.br; Av. Pedro de Toledo, 1800 – Vila Clementino, São Paulo – São Paulo – Brazil.

Introduction

Normal pressure hydrocephalus (NPH) is a neurological syndrome which manifests typically between 60 and 80 years of age, characterized by a triad of symptoms consisting of gait apraxia, dementia and urinary incontinence, associated with ventriculomegaly (detected radiologically) and normal pressure of the cerebrospinal fluid (CSF) [1-3].

NPH can be divided into two categories: idiopathic and secondary. The secondary NPH occurs in the context of neurological events such as subarachnoid hemorrhage (SAH), intraventricular hemorrhage caused by trauma or aneurysm rupture and meningitis. In contrast, idiopathic NPH usually occurs between the sixth and eighth decades of life and does not have its pathophysiological mechanisms completely understood [4-6]. Once NPH is a rare case of reversible dementia, it is essential to have an adequate clinical assessment, early diagnosis and proper treatment in such cases 4-7. Standard treatment is accomplished through the implantation of a ventricular shunt, offering the possibility of significant neurological improvement [7-9]. We briefly summarize main data about neuroimage in NPH, focusing in functional tests, differential diagnosis and predicition of shunt response.

Diagnostic Imaging

1. Computed Tomography (CT)

CT is a useful tool and still applicable in the evaluation of NPH, although magnetic resonance (MR) is the best image approach. It is usually a screening exam and main characteristics evaluated are dilated ventricles, disproportionate cortical atrophy and Evans index (Figure 1) [1-12].

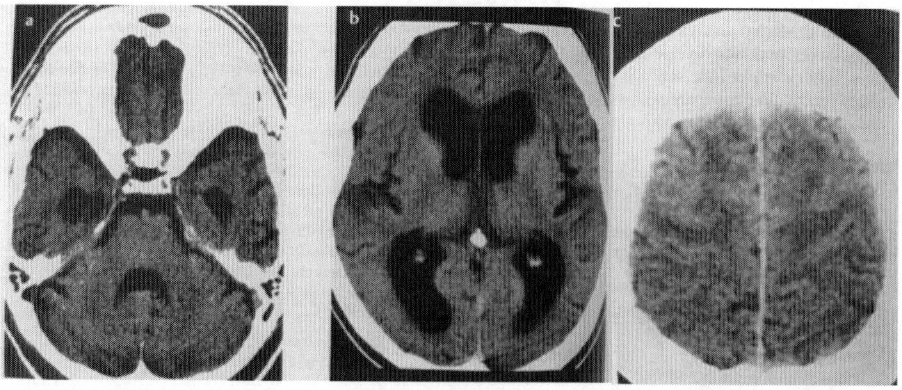

Figure 1. Typical CT in NPH: ventriculomegaly with cortical atrophy and loss of sulci in vertex.

2. Anatomical MR

MR imaging has several advantages over CT. At first, it is a more detailed anatomical examination, which may also be added to functional and metabolic evaluations. MR imaging is more sensitive than CT in depicting CSF spaces. Magnetic resonance is also attractive because of lack of radioation and noninvasive nature. In addition, idiopathic NPH may frequently affect the elderly, in whom these features may be associated with age-related brain atrophy [7-12].

The imaging signs of NPH include the distinctive morphologic changes of disproportionately dilated ventricles and a lack of cortical atrophy. The finding of an enlargement of the sylvian fissure and the basal cistern are also features of shunt-responsive idiopathic NPH. Other reported determinants of hydrocephalus severity on conventional cross sectional imaging include small cortical sulci (less than 1.9 mm) and periventricular hypodensity on CT or periventricular T2 hyperintensity on MR (Figure 2) [8,9,10].

MR can delineate changes in periventricular white matter, reveal the CSF flow void through the aqueduct and measure the volume of the CSFis the most powerful tool for the evaluation of this disorder. However, there has been no clear cut relationship between clinical improvement post-shunting and a decrease in ventriculomegaly. CSF flow void within the aqueduct greater than 18 mL/min suggests NPH [11,12].

NPH is often difficult to differentiate from degenerative and vascular dementias in older patients because of the occurrence of brain atrophy with ventricular dilatation, also called hydrocephalus ex vacuo or central atrophy [1-12].

Patients with NPH present usually with dilated ventricles and small parahippocampal fissures (PF), whereas patients with Alzheimer disease (AD) had dilated PF and ventricles that were enlarged but significantly smaller than those in patients with NPH. The findings regarding the PFs appear highly sensitive and specific, with very small overlap between the two groups (Figure 3) [12].

In patients with shunt-responsive idiopathic NPH, the CSF volume is significantly increased in all parts of the ventricular system as compared with those with Alzheimer disease or vascular dementia, whereas the superior convexity and medial subarachnoid CSF spaces were reduced tight suprasylvian subarachnoid spaces. All abnormalities of CSF distribution detected in idiopathic NPH were corrected with shunt surgery, indicating that these changes are related to NPH [9,10,11].

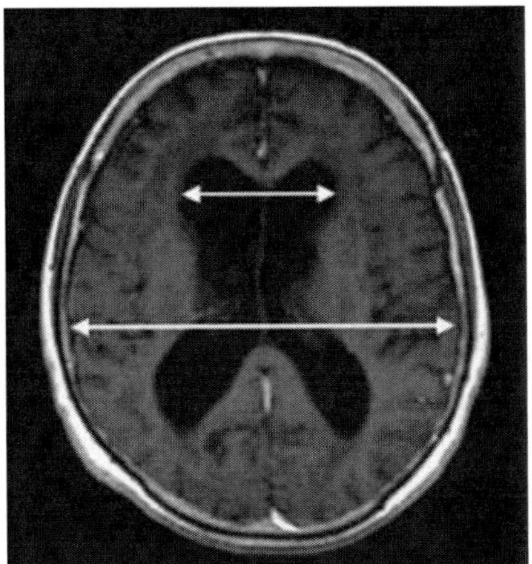

Figure 2. MR in NPH, displaying hydrocephalus and Evans Ratio.

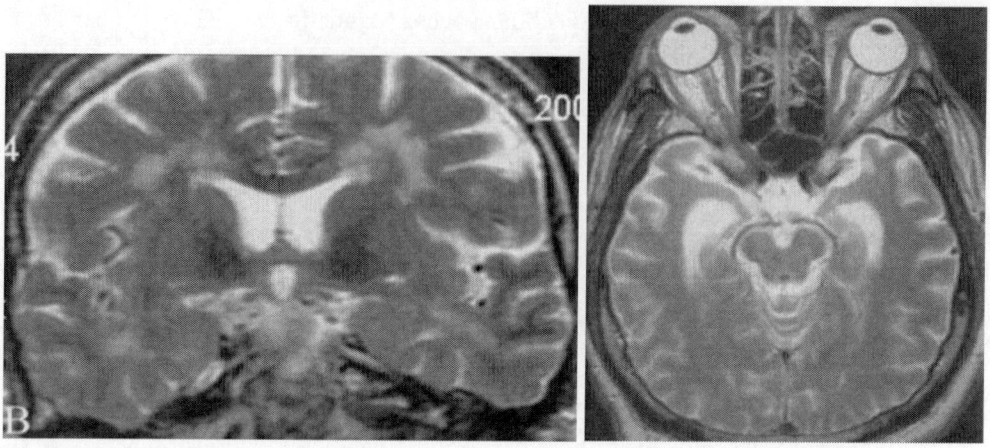

Figure 3. MR in differential diagnosis of NPH. At left, vascular dementia, with ventriculomegaly and periventricular hyperintensities in T2 suggesting previous vascular events. At right, ventriculomegaly and atrophy of hippocampus and parahyppocampal gyrus in Alzheimer Disease.

Measurement of the callosal angle (CA) on the coronal MR images of the posterior commissure perpendicular to the anteroposterior commissure plane may also be evaluated in NPH patients. CA in the NPH group (66 +/- 14 degrees) is significantly smaller than those of the Alzheimer Disease (104 +/- 15 degrees) and normal aging (112 +/- 11 degrees) groups [11].

However, definite morphologic features of idiopathic NPH remain undefined. No difference in the mean ventricular volume ratio, the mean brain volume ratio, the mean pericerebral CSF volume ratio, and the mean ratio between ventricular and pericerebral CSF volume is found between subjects who improved on gait or cognition or bladder function and those who did not [1-12].

3. Functional MR

Functional MR studies revealed improvement in motor functioning after CSF drainage related to improvement of high-order motor processes, rather than increased signalling from the primary motor cortex via the corticospinal tract, with enhancement of supplementary motor area [13].

Diffusion weighted image is also of value, once mean diffusion coefficient in the NPH group is usually higher than that in the ex vacuo ventricular dilatation and control groups. Patients with Alzheimer disease did not differ from ex vacuo dilatation patients and controls [12,13,14].

Cine Phase-Contrast MR

Cine phase-contrast MR quantifies CSF flow in terms of stroke volume, defined as mean volume of CSF passing through the cerebral aqueduct in systole and diastole. Stroke volume greater than 42 μL may predict the likelihood of response to VPS [12,13,14]. CSF stroke volume increases after onset of symptoms, reaches a plateau after 18 to 20 months and then declines, suggesting that increased flow associated with ventriculomegaly might cause shear stress on periventricular tissues that would be reversible with VPS. At this time, there is insufficient evidence to determine the value of this imaging technique in predicting response to shunting in iNPH, but an elevated CSF stroke volume is considered a supportive criterion for diagnosis (Figure 4) [12,13,14,15,16].

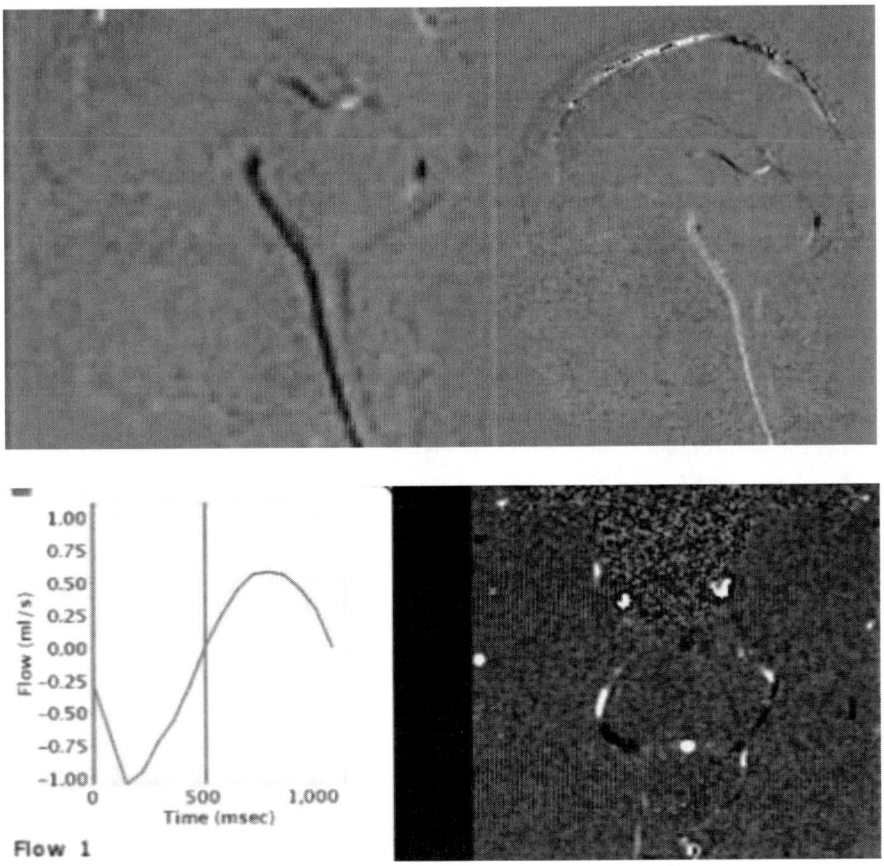

Figure 4. Flow study in MR.

4. MR Spectroscopy

Significant preoperative differences in N-acetyl aspartate (NAA)/creatine (Cr) and NAA/choline (Cho) may be noted between patients with excellent and poor outcome. Multiple regression analysis linked higher preoperative NAA/Cr ratio, gait score, and modified Rankin scale to better one month outcome. Multiple regression analysis indicated that NAA/Cho had the best predictive value for one year outcome [12,13,14].

5. Positron Emission Tomography (PET)

Pittsburgh compound B (PIB) PET presents with retention in patients with idiopathic normal pressure hydrocephalus (iNPH). PIB retention is limited to the high-convexity parasagittal areas in iNPH patients, whereas it spread over the frontal and parietotemporal areas in AD [16]. Cerebral blood flow (CBF) evaluated in NPH revealed that the white matter CBF is reduced in NPH, with an abnormal gradient from the lateral ventricles towards the subcortical white matter. Such reduced CBF appears to be maximal in the paraventricular watershed region. Metabolism rate, evaluated through cerebral metabolic rate (CMR), is also diffusely low [17,18]. After shunting, iNPH patients usually improved and CBF increases in all regions. These findings confirm that iNPH is a disease involving all cerebral regions almost in the same way, and shunt procedure has a similar effect on regional cerebral metabolism almost in the same way. Individual variations of CMRglu are more important than absolute values and correlate with clinical status after shunting. Clinical improvement depends not only on the capability to restore the cerebrospinal fluid dynamic, but also on the ability of cerebral parenchyma to recover the metabolic function [17,18].

6. Single Photon Emission Computed Tomography (SPECT)

Poor increase of CBF by acetazolamide implies a low capacity for vasodilation in the brain due to compression and stretching by ventriculomegaly. Acetazolamide SPECT study is not an absolute examination but one of the valuable supplementary objective examinations to determine the surgical indication in iNPH-suspected patients (Figure 5). There was a significant decrease in tracer activity in the right-side-dominant bilateral frontal cortex and the left inferior temporal gyrus in the severe urinary dysfunction group [19,20].

Urinary dysfunction was found to be closely related with right frontal hypoperfusion in iNPH using [(123) I]-IMP SPECT. This right frontal area is one of the critical areas for regulating micturition. While secondary incontinence can result from gait disturbance or dementia, there may also be a neurogenic mechanism underlying urinary dysfunction, which is a significant burden in patients with iNPH and their caregivers. There is also decreased blood flow around the corpus callosum and, in iNPH, enhanced perfusion in areas surrounding the cingulate gyrus in the sagittal view, while no Alzheimer Disease cases showed these findings [19,20].

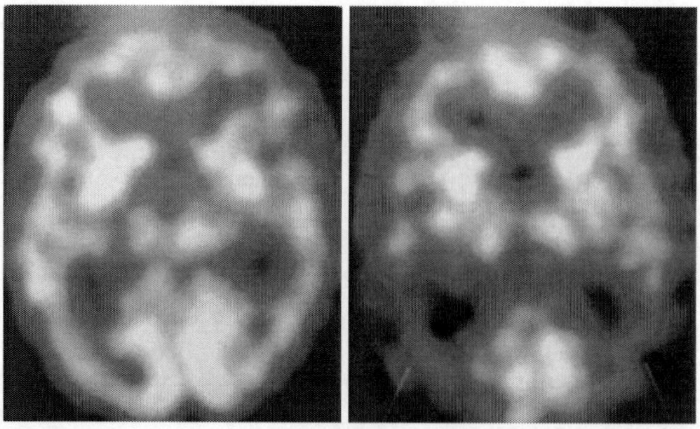

Figure 5. SPECT in differential diagnosis of NPH. At left, normal subject with preserved metabolism. At right, a subject with Alzheimer disease and decreased metabolism in associative cerebral areas.

7. Cisternography

Cisternography may be performed with Tomographic cisternography (CTC), radionuclide cisternography (RC) and magnetic resonance cisternography (MRC). Magnetic resonance cisternography has advantages which include the absence of radiation, high soft tissue resolution and capacity for multi-planar imaging. MRC is generally used to diagnose CSF fistulae and identify the communication of arachnoid cysts (ACs) with neighboring CSF areas by showing CSF dynamics [21,22].

Radionuclide cisternography seems to be the most physiological method that allows to gain more direct insight into the dynamics and the PM-R flow and its absorption. The results of the radioisotope examination turn out to be the most reliable criterion in the diagnostics of NPH [12,21,22].

MRC can evaluate the CSF circulation physiologically and can show a blockage in the CSF absorption if it exists. INPH patients usually present remaining contrast material in lateral ventricles at the 12th and 24th hours. No contrast material is present in the control cases at the 48th hour. The contrast material is significantly more prevalent in the INPH patients at the 24th and the 48th hours compared with the control cases. Such criteria for INPH are related to better response to shunt [19,20].

8. EEG

Unfortunately, conventional neuroimaging methods such as single photon emission computed tomography (SPECT) and functional magnetic resonance imaging (fMRI), as well as electroencephalogram (EEG) power analysis seem to have failed to detect the effect of CSF tapping on brain function [23].

Neuronal Activity Topography (NAT) analysis, which calculates normalized power variance (NPV) of EEG waves, to detect cortical functional changes induced by CSF tapping in iNPH NAT analysis can detect CSF tapping-induced functional changes in cortical activity, in a way that no other neuroimaging methods have been able to do so far, and can predict clinical response to shunt operation in patients with iNPH. After Tap test, it was observed decrease in alpha NPV at the medial frontal cortex in shunt responders, while nonresponders exhibited an increase in alpha NPV at the right dorsolateral prefrontal cortex [23].

9. Hemodynamics Studies

Hemodynamic evaluation may be performed with vascular functional examination. Cerebral blood flow (CBF) and vascular response to acetazolamide can be assessed through xenon-enhanced computed tomography. Preoperatively, NPH patients had globally reduced CBF, but the reduction was more pronounced in those who did not improve after shunt. The vascular response was impaired only in the white matter of the patients who improved later. After shunting, restoration of CBF, more marked in the white matter, and recovery of vascular response in the white matter paralleled clinical improvement and a reduction in ventricular dilation and periventricular lucency on computed tomographic scans. The CBF reduction, however, deteriorated in patients who did not improve clinically [13,14,15,24,25].

Underlying disease in the improved patients was ischemia, with a loss of autoregulatory capacity in the periventricular white matter caused by cerebrospinal fluid diffusion. Those who did not improve had irreversible brain damage in which the CBF reduction was secondary to metabolic depression and autoregulation was preserved. We also conclude that patients suspected of having NPH will improve clinically after shunting if preoperative hemispheric CBF is greater than 20 ml/100 g per minute and the vascular response to acetazolamide is impaired only in the periventricular white matter. They will not improve, however, if the preoperative CBF is less than 20 ml/100 g per minute and the vascular response to acetazolamide is intact [24,25].

Studying the relationship between cerebral hemodynamics and clinical performance in NPH before and after surgery our data suggest that higher cerebral blood flow velocity before surgery in patients with NPH is related to clinical improvement after shunt surgery. Cerebral hemodynamic parameters may develop into predictors of successful shunt surgery in patients with NPH [24,25].

Conclusion

Diagnosis and treatment of normal pressure hydrocephalus remains unclear despite the development of guidelines. Once NPH is a rare case of reversible dementia, it is essential to have an adequate clinical assessment, early diagnosis and proper treatment in such cases.

Several different clinical trials have evidence heterogeneous results due to heterogeneity in study protocols and lack of a universally accepted standard in NPH management.

Neuroimage is a fundamental tool to perform differential diagnosis with normal aging, Alzheimer disease and other types of dementia. Together with clinical status, it is the main instrument to predict shunt response. Functional and metabolic studies are increasingly being added to diagnoses apparatus, due to their sensivity and specificity, however they are still expensive and sometimes applied only in research protocols.

References

[1] Hakim S, Adams RD. The special clinical problem of symptomatic hydrocephalus with normal cerebrospinal fluid pressure: observations on cerebrospinal fluid hydrodynamics. *J. Neurol. Sci.* 1965;2: 307–327.

[2] Adams RD, Fisher CM, Hakim S, Ojemann RG, Sweet WH. Symptomatic occult hydrocephalus with "normal" cerebrospinal fluid pressure: a treatable syndrome. *N. Engl. J. Med.* 1965;273:117– 126.

[3] Katzman R. Normal pressure hydrocephalus. In: Wells CE, ed. Dementia. 2nd ed. Philadelphia: F.A. Davis; 1977:69–92.

[4] Vanneste JA, Augstijn P, Dirven C, Tan WF, Goedhart ZD. Shunting normal-pressure hydrocephalus: do the benefits outweigh the risks? A multicenter study and literature review. *Neurology* 1992; 42:54–59.

[5] Wikkelso C, Andersson H, Blomstrand C, Matousek M, Svendsen P. Computed tomography of the brain in the diagnosis of and prognosis in normal pressure hydrocephalus. *Neuroradiology* 1989; 31:160–165.
[6] George AE. Chronic communicating hydrocephalus and periventricular white matter disease: a debate with regard to cause and effect. *AJNR Am. J. Neuroradiol.* 1991;12:42–44.
[7] Sasaki M, Honda S, Yuasa T, Iwamura A, Shibata E, Ohba H. Narrow CSF space at high convexity and high midline areas in idiopathic normal pressure hydrocephalus detected by axial and coronal MRI. *Neuroradiology.* 2008 Feb;50(2):117-22.
[8] Adachi M, Kawanami T, Ohshima F, Kato T. Upper midbrain profile sign and cingulate sulcus sign: MRI findings on sagittal images in idiopathic normal-pressure hydrocephalus, Alzheimer's disease, and progressive supranuclear palsy. *Radiat. Med.* 2006 Oct;24(8):568-72.
[9] Bradley WG Jr, Bahl G, Alksne JF. Idiopathic normal pressure hydrocephalus may be a "two hit" disease: benign external hydrocephalus in infancy followed by deep white matter ischemia in late adulthood. *J. Magn Reson Imaging.* 2006 Oct;24(4):747-55.
[10] Moghekar A, Rigamonti D. Neuroradiological diagnosis of idiopathic normal-pressure hydrocephalus: the search for the Holy Grail. *Ann. Neurol.* 2009 Oct;66(4):436-7.
[11] Ishii K, Kanda T, Harada A, Miyamoto N, Kawaguchi T, Shimada K, Ohkawa S, Uemura T, Yoshikawa T, Mori E. Clinical impact of the callosal angle in the diagnosis of idiopathic normal pressure hydrocephalus. Eur Radiol. 2008 Nov;18(11):2678-83.
[12] Mori K: Management of idiopathic normal-pressure hydrocephalus: a multiinstitutional study conducted in Japan. *J. Neurosurg.* 95:970–973, 2001.
[13] Lenfeldt N, Larsson A, Nyberg L, Andersson M, Birgander R, Eklund A, Malm J.Idiopathic normal pressure hydrocephalus: increased supplementary motor activity accounts for improvementafter CSF drainage. *Brain.* 2008 Nov;131(Pt 11):2904-12.
[14] Ng SE, Low AM, Tang KK, Chan YH, Kwok RK. Value of quantitative MRI biomarkers (Evans' index, aqueductal flow rate, and apparent diffusion coefficient) in idiopathic normal pressure hydrocephalus. *J. Magn Reson Imaging.* 2009 Oct;30(4):708-15.
[15] Calcagni ML, Taralli S, Mangiola A, Indovina L, Lavalle M, De Bonis P, Anile C, Giordano A. Regional cerebral metabolic rate of glucose evaluation and clinical assessment in patients with idiopathic normal-pressure hydrocephalus before and after ventricular shunt placement: a prospective analysis. *Clin. Nucl. Med.* 2013 Jun;38(6):426-31.
[16] Kondo M, Tokuda T, Itsukage M, Kuriyama N, Matsushima S, Yamada K, Nakanishi H, Ishikawa M, Nakagawa M. Distribution of amyloid burden differs between idiopathic normal pressure hydrocephalus and Alzheimer's disease. *Neuroradiol. J.* 2013 Feb;26(1):41-6.
[17] Yamada SM, Masahira N, Kawanishi Y, Fujimoto Y, Shimizu K. Preoperative acetazolamide SPECT is useful for predicting outcome of shunt operation in idiopathicnormal pressure hydrocephalus patients. *Clin. Nucl. Med.* 2013 Sep;38(9):671-6.
[18] Sakakibara R, Uchida Y, Ishii K, Kazui H, Hashimoto M, Ishikawa M, Yuasa T, Kishi M, Ogawa E, Tateno F, Uchiyama T, Yamamoto T, Yamanishi T, Terada H;SINPHONI (Study of Idiopathic Normal Pressure Hydrocephalus On Neurological

Improvement). Correlation of right frontal hypoperfusion and urinary dysfunction in iNPH: a SPECT study. *Neurourol. Urodyn.* 2012 Jan;31(1):50-5.

[19] Nakayama T, Ouchi Y, Yoshikawa E, Sugihara G, Torizuka T, Tanaka K. Striatal D2 receptor availability after shunting in idiopathic normal pressure hydrocephalus. *J. Nucl. Med.* 2007 Dec;48(12):1981-6.

[20] Kobayashi S, Tateno M, Utsumi K, Takahashi A, Morii H, Saito T. Two-layer appearance on brain perfusion SPECT in idiopathic normal pressure hydrocephalus: a qualitative analysis by using easy Z-score imaging system, eZIS. *Dement Geriatr Cogn Disord.* 2009;28(4):330-7.

[21] Enzmann DR, Norman D, Price DC, Newton TH. Metrizamide and radionuclide cisternography in communicating hydrocephalus. *Radiology* 1979;130:681–686 12.

[22] Chmielowski K, Podgórski JK, Twarkowski P, Pietrzykowski J, Szaluś N. Radionuclide cisternography in the diagnosis of normal pressure hydrocephalus. *Pol. Merkur Lekarski.* 2004 Jun;16(96):576-80.

[23] Aoki Y, Kazui H, Tanaka T, Ishii R, Wada T, Ikeda S, Hata M, Canuet L, Musha T, Matsuzaki H, Imajo K, Yoshiyama K, Yoshida T, Shimizu Y, Nomura K, Iwase M, Takeda M. EEG and Neuronal Activity Topography analysis can predict effectiveness of shunt operation in idiopathic normal pressure hydrocephalus patients. *Neuroimage Clin.* 2013 Oct 19;3:522-30.

[24] Chen YF, Wang YH, Hsiao JK, Lai DM, Liao CC, Tu YK, Liu HM. Normal pressure hydrocephalus: cerebral hemodynamic, metabolism measurement, discharge score, and long-term outcome. *Surg. Neurol.* 2008 Dec;70 Suppl 1:S1:69-77; discussion S1:77.

[25] Bakker SL, Boon AJ, Wijnhoud AD, Dippel DW, Delwel EJ, Koudstaal PJ. Cerebral hemodynamics before and after shunting in normal pressure hydrocephalus. *Acta Neurol. Scand.* 2002 Sep;106(3):123-7.

Index

A

B

C

D

E

F

G

H

I

N

O

P

Q

R

S

T

U

V

W

X

Y